Public Health and Politics in the Age of Reform

Public Health and Politics in the Age of Reform: Cholera, the State and the Royal Navy in Victorian Britain

David McLean

BLOOMSBURY ACADEMIC
LONDON • NEW YORK • OXFORD • NEW DELHI • SYDNEY

BLOOMSBURY ACADEMIC
Bloomsbury Publishing Plc
50 Bedford Square, London, WC1B 3DP, UK
1385 Broadway, New York, NY 10018, USA

BLOOMSBURY, BLOOMSBURY ACADEMIC and the Diana
logo are trademarks of Bloomsbury Publishing Plc

First published in Great Britain by I.B. Tauris 2006
Paperback edition published by Bloomsbury Academic 2020

A catalogue record for this book is available from the British Library.

A catalog record for this book is available from the Library of Congress.

ISBN: HB: 978-1-8451-1069-7
PB: 978-1-3501-7617-1
ePDF: 978-0-8577-1596-8
eBook: 978-0-7556-2055-1

Series: International Library of Historical Studies, vol. 33

Typeset by ITS, Edinburgh

To find out more about our authors and books visit
www.bloomsbury.com and sign up for our newsletters.

Contents

Acknowledgements

I am grateful for the Small Grants in Humanities from King's College, London which contributed towards travel costs and to my wife, Eva Gordon, for her continuing support and constructive advice.

Introduction

MANY FRACTURES RUN deep across the landscape of public health, local government and the ever-increasing role of centralised authority in modern Britain. For some participants in this historical debate, and the more so for those who would select from it for political advantage, ideology and accepted social wisdom can be uncomfortably challenged by too much attention to the details of the past. All applaud the fact that the health and longevity of Britain's population improved after the early nineteenth century. How that improvement came about, however, is more controversial, calling into question, as it does, the contribution of expanded state machinery as against the effects of rising economic prosperity stemming from the natural interplay of market forces. McKeown's work of the 1960s and 1970s disturbed the liberal consensus about heroic medicine and beneficent planners by asserting that the impact of human intervention was statistically marginal in a population now sufficiently nourished.[1] The past is easily clouded by opinions held about the present.

Worse still, the past can take on a function: knowledge of the nineteenth century is filtered through a prism designed to interpret developments in the next and thereby falls prey to those who seek evolutionary traces of the world around them.[2] Despite paying lip service to the past as different, academic tracts too often suggest simply that failure to adopt the practices of a later age resulted from an ubiquitous mixture of exploitative commercial interests, inadequate laws and outdated administrative structures. Of course, none of these need apply. A common vocabulary across the generations does not denote a similar culture: the application of law and the remit of authority exist within their intellectual and social environments. Furthermore, the concept of good legislation is highly subjective and most profitably defined perhaps as that which is implementable rather than that which expresses lofty ideals realisable only far in the future, if at all. Understanding that is prerequisite for work in the field. High-minded aristocrats, radical politicians, careerist officials, medical experts and parliamentary draftsmen moved in circles where principled debate may well have provided a common currency, but these were not usually the circles of magistrates or local administrators who frequently struggled with ideas and legal language which did not translate easily into the real world. Implementing well-meant but imprecise legislation caused difficulties. A court action where costs would be high, where the burden of proof weighed heavily upon prosecutors and claimants and where a successful outcome might have a damaging effect on a locality's economy and the livelihoods of ordinary people often made judgment, let alone subsequent enforcement, a far cry from the wording of statute. In early-nineteenth-century Britain the law was assumed to protect the freedoms of people and their property – not to proscribe them. That others might suffer thereby was a lesser evil.

Not only has the engine for nineteenth-century health improvement proved contentious, but the pace of change has also been questioned. The idea of a revolution in government has suggested identifiable years of accelerated progress.[3] Likewise, the study of nineteenth-century epidemics, particularly cholera, can suggest that natural calamities served as stimuli for uneven advances in public health. Increased sickness and mortality were doubtless forceful: in times of crisis advocates of reform would always find the general mood more receptive to the encroachments of public authorities.[4] Yet this approach risks losing sight of slower and less dramatic change. The nineteenth century witnessed a continuing struggle between the rights of private property and concerns about the cost to society of widespread poverty, much of which was arguably reinforced by the debilitating effects of disease. Epidemics certainly maintained momentum; they were not necessarily, however, instigators of change.

The same might be said of Acts of Parliament. These have long attracted attention because they reassure proponents of state endeavour and because they conform more readily to accounts of national history. But the history of public health is not perhaps a history best viewed in national terms. Nineteenth-century Parliaments sometimes enabled but rarely provided. The history of public health is more plausibly the history of local events and local government. It was at provincial level that political engagement could be at its fiercest and from where the impetus and, crucially, the money had to come. Local government remained important in Britain throughout the nineteenth century. While municipal autonomy may well be charged with obstructing pressures from London for sanitary improvement until the 1860s, thereafter civic pride could also act as a spur for the large capital projects eventually undertaken. Local politics were not just scaled-down squabbles about national issues but had vibrancy and an agenda of their own, with electoral outcomes often diverging from the fortunes of the parties at Westminster.

Needless to say, therefore, trying to construct an aggregate pattern for public health improvement can dissolve into a frustrating exercise for those who strive for a nationwide framework for historical enquiry. Broad assumptions and conclusions appear as mirages always retreating beyond a foreground cluttered with local studies all pointing the traveller in different directions. But if cities, boroughs and rural districts responded at a varying pace to a range of problems, adopted statutory procedures at different times, operated according to their peculiar political and administrative customs usually enshrined in ancient legislation, and when Justices set new laws against existing Acts or ruled as they felt best suited immediate circumstances, then the search for a single history may be ever unrewarded.

But the study of specific communities does not acquire merit merely by default. While such work tests the patience of scholars who prefer broad sweeps, local investigations impose the discipline of chronology and narrative which determine cause and effect and which demonstrate the practical contributions of individuals and institutions to their society. In their proper context, as Keith Wrightson has observed, local studies 'can do much to make concrete and accessible the abstractions and generalisations of historical interpretation'.[5] It is also at provincial level that the most telling sources may exist – even if they do not always lead researchers where they most wish to go. Reviewing Hilary Marland's major work on medicine and society in Yorkshire towns, John Pickstone laments at one point that the analysis or research material could not be fuller.[6] Exploring interactions and confrontations within regional communities can indeed, as he insists, throw considerable light upon the tensions which might either advance or retard the cause of public health, provided, of course, that their inhabitants leave sufficient clues behind. Survival of the records is an inevitable hazard of the historian's trade. What follows here none the less represents a remarkable survival in both parochial and private archives and, most unusually, at the Admiralty, revealing experiments and developments in public health and the upheavals which occurred in local government amid the chaos of a devastating epidemic along the south Devon coast in the 1840s.

CHAPTER 1

Disease, Politics and Poverty in Nineteenth-century Britain

WHEN THE GERMAN scientist Robert Koch identified the cholera bacillus in 1884 he ended a debate which had divided medical opinion in Europe for over half a century. A micro-organism which multiplied in a warm and humid environment was now proven to be the cause of the epidemics which had swept across the continent since the early 1830s. The symptoms and severity of cholera had been known since its discovery in Bengal in 1816; furthermore, it had long been associated with contaminated food and water and with the squalor so characteristic of Europe's growing cities. But was it contagious or infectious? On this there was no agreement: copious and persuasive evidence was marshalled by proponents of both points of view. And even if it were transferred by human contact, the means by which this was done could not be demonstrated. Miasmatic theories remained strong in nineteenth-century medical discourse. Foul air was not simply a warning that disease might be festering but was itself the carrier of unknown agents which struck down those predisposed by weakness or by personal neglect. Until the 1860s germs were but concepts and bacteriology was an unimaginable branch of science. Nevertheless, by observation, deduction and attention to the rudiments of public health it was possible to contain the ravages of cholera without being able precisely to define it. Britain experienced no significant outbreak after 1866. Other parts of Europe, however, were less fortunate. As late as 1892 cholera claimed more than 8,000 lives in Hamburg – 13 per cent of the city's population. Identifying the cause and preventing the occurrence, of course, were not the same.[1]

There was no cure for what was widely referred to as Asiatic cholera, nor any consensus as to the most effective treatment. In many cases the opportunity for treatment never arose. Once in the digestive tract the bacillus bred rapidly, causing a huge loss of body fluid and, in its severest form, death within hours. The speed with which even the strong and healthy could be reduced to prostration was among the most alarming features of the disease. The poor, herded together amid the grime of urban Britain, were, as with most diseases, particularly susceptible, though given the varied means by which it was transmitted cholera afflicted all classes of society and could produce panic in the face of epidemic not seen in Britain since the late seventeenth century. Uncertainty of cause and the swiftness of demise then combined with the nature of the illness to make cholera so feared. Death by uncontrollable vomiting and emissions was a distressing end and whole families and households could be struck down together. The bacillus was in all bodily discharges and was passed on via unwashed hands, infected clothing and flies. Once in the population the chief defence was strict personal hygiene. This much was surmised as early as the 1830s. Some who studied the disease were convinced even then that its source lay in the unwholesome water supply in many towns and cities, the population merely drawing back from rivers effluence which had been introduced upstream.

Acclaimed as Koch was, the Italian Filippo Pacini was later accredited with the discovery of the bacillus in research published in 1854. In the same year empirical research demonstrated that water, by whatever mechanism, was the principal distributor of cholera. At the height of one epidemic John Snow observed the remarkable correlation between the spread of cholera in London and the supply of water from a specific pump. When the pump was closed down the disease at once abated.[2] Snow published these observations and an extensive and compelling study of infection within the supply zone of the Lambeth Water Company, but he could not prove the connection. Proven or not, water remained a major concern for Victorian public health reformers; an unpolluted supply by properly managed companies was a matter not only for local political debate but one of national significance when applied to London. Of course, aspirations for reform extended further than providing clean water. By the middle decades of the nineteenth century much educated opinion in Britain had come to recognise the dangers caused by precipitant urban growth. Vast towns and cities now served an economy largely transformed from agricultural to industrial production. In 1801 only 20 per cent of the population of England and Wales had lived in towns with a population above 5,000; by 1851 that figure had soared to 54 per cent and the largest ten urban centres now contained a quarter of the nation's population. At the beginning of the century only London could boast a population above 100,000 persons. By 1851 that of Liverpool was 376,000, Glasgow 345,000, Manchester 303,000, Birmingham 233,000, Edinburgh 194,000, Leeds 172,000, Bristol 137,000, Sheffield 135,000 and Bradford 104,000. By the early 1850s London's population stood at 2.5 million. The landscape of Britain and the distribution of its people had altered within the span of one generation. For the majority, however, the social infrastructure of housing, policing, education and public health lagged far behind the revolutionary advances in transport and manufacturing technology.[3]

Victorian society lived with the ever-present threat of disease. Even so, Britain's four cholera epidemics of 1831–32, 1848–49, 1853–54 and 1866 were the sharpest reminders of life's transitory nature and certainly caused the greatest hysteria. About 31,000 died from cholera in mainland Britain in 1831–32 with a further 21,000 in Ireland. The 1848–49 outbreak carried off over 62,000 of whom 53,000 were in England alone. 23,000 died in 1853–54, almost half of whom lived in London. In 1866 the death toll was 14,000 nationwide. Regional concentrations undoubtedly increased the impact in the areas worst affected. Inexplicably both London and Birmingham largely escaped in 1831–32. In 1849 Hull was the worst-affected city with more than 2,000 deaths from a population of only 80,000. Liverpool lost well over 5,000 from among its 300,000 inhabitants. Horrifying too was the high incidence of mortality. Untended, up to 60 per cent of cases might prove fatal. Treatment, when available, could improve the chances of survival, but once the patient had been weakened and collapse occurred the outcome was widely held to be inevitable.

Cholera was not the nineteenth century's greatest killer. Smallpox, typhus, influenza, diphtheria and tuberculosis scythed through Britain's population, although their progress seemed less spectacular and certainly lacked the shock effect of a cholera epidemic. Tuberculosis, in fact, accounted for one-third of all deaths from disease in the Victorian period, claiming 59,000 victims in 1838 alone. Smallpox killed 42,000 people in Britain in the outbreak of 1837–40 and influenza swept away 50,000 in London in 1847–48. In the late 1840s and early 1850s deaths both from typhus and from diarrhoea were comparable with the toll exacted by the Asiatic cholera epidemic, but cholera, like nothing else, focused the Victorian consciousness on the state of health of the masses and on the hopelessly inadequate city infrastructure which so fouled the air, rivers and streets of those towering symbols of economic progress within the poorer quarters of which so many of Britain's inhabitants now eked out their miserable lives.[4] The wealthier classes began to move to more salubrious suburbs. Meanwhile the resources of the state and of local government were gradually but increasingly employed legislating and providing for a better environment – ultimately, campaigners argued, for the sake of all.

Cholera exposed not only the parameters of scientific discovery and the dangers of neglect in public health: its epidemics revealed also the limits of medical care in the nineteenth century. Many practitioners claimed that they could cure cholera and there were a variety of published accounts, each reporting unprecedented rates of success. Some extolled the virtue of saline solutions given to replenish the body's loss of fluid and salts. In desperation a saline solution might even be injected intravenously after collapse had occurred. Most treatments involved purging the intestines of morbid agents; this would not only cleanse the digestive system but in doing so reactivate a vigorous circulation of the blood. Castor oil with calomel were favoured purgatives. Calming the patient in order to bring down fever and to ameliorate intestinal cramps and muscular spasms by which fluid was lost was also deemed essential. Opium was thus administered as a sedative in many cases. Brandy, wine and tea were usually given when the patient was able to hold liquids. Different hospitals had preferred variations of these remedies, although most surgeons or physicians candidly admitted that nuances in treatment were not important. In fact the treatments prescribed barely changed between 1831 and 1866.[5] The most important aid was likely to be basic nursing. Keeping a patient warm, clean and reasonably comfortable and replacing fluids when possible were generally accepted as the best that medical training could provide. If such care reached the sick in time and was conscientiously applied, then what began as a severe diarrhoea might be contained as such or else progress no further than what was frequently described as choleraic diarrhoea. From this, recovery after convalescence was normal. Blurred distinctions between diarrhoea, choleraic diarrhoea and full-blown Asiatic cholera often made the claims of medical men and quacks hard to judge.[6] Special cures and near-miraculous medicines were always available to a public willing to believe and buy almost anything in times of crisis.

Reflecting on the spread of a new epidemic across the country in February 1849, one newspaper declared emphatically that 'it is more easy to prevent than cure an attack of cholera'.[7] This was both scientifically true and by now the loud cry of a generation of social and administrative reformers convinced that only a widespread overhaul of water, sewerage and drainage facilities, legislative change and a modernisation of those authorities responsible for the nation's public health could possibly tackle the root cause of so much disease in mid-nineteenth-century Britain. This was sensitive ground to tread. It was easy to reach agreement about the merits of medical discovery. Such advance was part of the technological wonder which so characterised the Victorian age; all would applaud a cure devised or a new surgical operation performed as a benefit to humanity and the fruit of a society which valued innovation. But it was also accepted wisdom that progress was achieved by individual enterprise amid unrestrained economic and social forces. Identifying groups whose distress might be the product of other than their own shortcomings and for whose failings a wider society and its regulatory structures might be, at least in part, to blame was not only to challenge assumptions of a natural order but to give succour to dangerous political ideologies which advocated a redistribution of both wealth and power. The poor were as they were for reasons of their own making and only by their own diligence could they raise themselves from the state into which they had fallen. To argue for a wider responsibility on the part of those who held power or who paid taxes was well-meaning but it infringed the freedom of others and threatened the stability of society by encouraging the lower orders to look to the state to compensate them for their own moral defects.

Yet by the 1840s such arguments were being advanced with some tangible rewards. Whether inspired by personal humanitarianism or by Benthamite images of a society safer when acting as an organic whole, a new generation of public servants, medical professionals and social reformers had come to see a betterment of communal health as a just cause which overrode the identity of the individual and the family. A right to create filth and to propagate pestilence might well enshrine the ancient liberties of every free-born Briton, but when the pestilence spread beyond the boundaries of his property then the liberties of others to live in comfort were violated. The idea grew that it was a necessary function of the state to hold the ring in this ideological clash between the real rights of the one and the collective, though often notional, rights of the many and that the means for so doing was parliamentary legislation empowering responsible bodies to act in the public good. Such legislation would follow open enquiry and be based on scientific evidence and expert opinion. Any legislation was bound to be controversial. The political motives of many reformers were questioned and their self-righteous delivery of what others regarded as at best quasi-scientific assertions was branded as intellectual arrogance. Championing the role of government in regulating the lives of its citizens was equally contentious. To trample down the sanctity of individual freedom, however distasteful some freedom might be, was inevitably to concentrate more power in the hands of a political elite. It opened a door for the expansion of centralised state authority and even for a descent into tyranny.

One man, Edwin Chadwick, seemed to provide a focus for this debate. Chadwick was a public official, not a politician, but his writings and his influence in Whig circles made him a hero for all who campaigned for reform in the early-Victorian era, while he was reviled as a manipulative, officious megalomaniac by those of a more cautious disposition.[8] Born in 1800 and educated in the Law, Chadwick began his career as Jeremy Bentham's secretary in 1831 and then assisted the nine Royal Commissioners appointed to investigate the Poor Laws in 1832. At this stage Chadwick's influence was largely unofficial and he enjoyed no political patronage. But he soon proved himself to be an industrious and able administrator, confident when handling voluminous data and combining them with a persuasive philosophy. When the Poor Law Commission was created in 1834 Chadwick was appointed Secretary, conducting much of its business in that capacity until 1847. His influence in government, however, went well beyond routine administration. Chadwick compiled and interpreted statistics in order to make the case for health reform. His work was aided by the creation of the Registrar General's Office in 1837, most notably by the data gathered there by the statistician William Farr after 1839. Farr, like many reformers, was eager to demonstrate a correlation between low living standards and the incidence of disease.[9] The Statistical Society of London and progressive medical practitioners likewise provided Chadwick with essential material for his crusade.

In 1837–38 a typhus epidemic in east London presented an opportunity to investigate sanitation in the area and to develop a subtle line of argument whereby the expense of improvements might be justified even to the unbelieving. The outbreak had come to the attention of the Poor Law Commissioners only because it had triggered a dramatic rise in the demand for poor relief. Furthermore, the parishes of east London had been obliged to commit large sums to removing accumulations of waste and prosecuting negligent landlords. Would it not be cheaper, Chadwick suggested, to prevent so much pauperism by eradicating the sickness which gave rise to it? A medical report on London typhus was published in 1839, followed by the wider investigation of the Health of Towns Select Committee of the House of Commons chaired by Robert Slaney in 1840. Chadwick's real rise to prominence came in 1842 with the appearance of his *Report on the Sanitary Condition of the Labouring Population of Great Britain*. It was a monumental study in which the author broadened his case for the role of the state as the arbiter of public health, using both scientific data and the accounts of scores of medical officers extracted from Poor Law reports. The 1842 *Report* sold over 100,000 copies. Drains, sewers, dirt and disease were henceforth not only matters of public awareness but rising higher on the political agenda. It was a milestone in the history of public health in Britain. Chadwick followed this with a report on the highly emotive issue of interments and burial practices in 1843.

Even Chadwick's admirers conceded that he was a difficult man with whom to work. Tactless, high-handed, uncompromising and self-opinionated, he was also easy prey for opponents, both in Whitehall and in the provinces, who resented his centralising inclinations. But by 1847 a momentum for public health provision had been achieved and Chadwick had extended his expertise further to the Health of Towns Royal Commission, the reports of which he largely wrote and produced in 1844 and 1845. Pressure for sanatory improvement in Britain was also stimulated at grassroots level by the Health of Towns Association, founded in London in December 1844 but within three years with thirteen branches in most major urban centres.[10] Though a purely voluntary movement, the Health of Towns Association brought together clergy, medical experts and local and even national political figures and it did much in the mid-1840s to disseminate knowledge and to educate public opinion at large on the relationship between squalor and disease. Public meetings were organised, pamphlets printed, the Liverpool and Plymouth Associations produced local publications, and the movement nationally issued the *Journal of Public Health and Monthly Record of Sanitary Improvement* in 1847 and 1848. Diverse as its membership was, all were happy to campaign for legislation which would create statutory authorities to address the problems so apparent in their towns. A victim of its own success, perhaps, the Health of Towns Association faded away in 1849. Its mission was largely accomplished when the first Nuisances Removal and Diseases Prevention Act passed through Parliament in 1846 and even more so when the Whig ministry of Lord John Russell implemented first a comprehensive Public Health Act in August 1848 and then a further Nuisances Removal Act just one month later.

London was exempted from this 1848 legislation: it was widely accepted that the scale of the capital's problems merited specific provision. On leaving the Poor Law Commission in 1847 Chadwick was given charge of the Metropolitan Sanitary Commission to enquire into London's ills and was an influential member of the Metropolitan Sewers Commission, established by a separate Act of Parliament, until 1849. Chadwick was now at the height of his career and his role in shaping public health policy was both recognised and formalised when, with Lord Ashley and Dr Thomas Southwood-Smith, he joined the General Board of Health created by the 1848 Public Health Act. There he was locked in a daily struggle against official indifference. 'We get no assistance but quiet hindrances from other offices,' he confided a year later. 'We are in continual conflict with the Treasury for advances of money.'[11] But he remained at the General Board of Health until removed in 1854.[12] Chadwick's work across twenty years helped overcome both inertia and resistance in making Britain's towns and cities better ventilated, better drained and more conscious of the need both to organise rudimentary medical services and to discharge sewage in such a way that the water supply ceased to be endangered. His efforts were instrumental in lessening the likelihood of epidemics and gradually increasing life expectancy. With a different temperament he might have achieved yet more. The hostility he attracted, almost needlessly at times, did exclude him from official bodies where his experience might have been of benefit but where his perceived enthusiasm for radically inspired central authority made his presence a political liability and ran the risk of institutional dysfunctionality. Lord Carlisle, First Commissioner of Woods, Forests and Land Revenue in 1849 with ministerial responsibility for the newly formed General Board of Health, was certainly aware of Chadwick's reputation. Appointing investigators for a further study of public health, Carlisle confessed to Russell as Prime Minister that 'I feel reluctantly bound to give in to the opinion that on the whole it may be most safe and prudent to leave Chadwick out of the new Commission'. 'At the same time,' he admitted, 'I still hold to the conviction that he knows more about the matter in hand than anyone else.'[13] Chadwick remained active in the cause which so dominated his life long after the end of his official career in 1854. By 1890, when he died, the role and power of the state in regulating the living conditions of its citizens had been transformed beyond recognition.

The reforming impulse of the 1830s and 1840s was by no means confined to improving health and sanitation. Political change was also in the air and the parliamentary reform of 1832 gave vitality to those who dreamed of recasting British society and its aristocratic institutions by demonstrating that even the constitution was not beyond their reach. The ensuing general election brought in a Whig ministry and a House of Commons committed to further legislation, a prime object of which was local government. In 1833 a Royal Commission was set up to investigate the outdated practices of municipal corporations and suitable men were appointed to ensure that there could be only one verdict. Despite the efficiency of some old corporations, such as those which administered King's Lynn and Wisbech,[14] the medieval and corrupt nature of local government was duly exposed and an Act designed to remedy its defects sped through Parliament in 1835. The Act was predicated on two basic assumptions: that local government had lost contact with the people and that the people wished it to be otherwise. Many, of course, did; the Municipal Corporations Act stipulated 178 boroughs where democracy among ratepayers would now supersede vested interest as the means of determining who held power in Britain's town halls.

It was hard to refute the view that the huge increase in urban populations in the early nineteenth century had created crises with which ancient structures of authority had never been designed to cope. The old municipal corporations owed their status to Royal Charters which had conferred upon merchant communities rights to regulate economic activity and to raise revenue from the inhabitants with which to maintain the basic infrastructure of small towns and their immediate environs. Corporations were empowered to make the rules by which townsmen lived; their officers acted as magistrates in order to ensure compliance. Within its area of jurisdiction a corporation was powerful, but beyond the pageantry of municipal office that power was invariably tempered by a restricted range of functions actually performed. In practice, while a corporation might own and administer the institutions of a town, it frequently did little which touched the daily lives of ordinary people. Municipal corporations held title to property as behoved private bodies, they were trustees of the grammar school and other charities, they granted market licences and maintained bridges within their boundaries. They also employed constables and watchmen and had a responsibility for the streets and repairing drainage. The essential privilege of a Royal Charter was that of urban self-government, free and distinct therefore from the county magistrates and nobility who controlled legal and administrative authority across the expanse of surrounding countryside and who usually knew and cared nothing for the separate culture and economic needs of town life. A Charter also conferred a separate parliamentary representation which by the late seventeenth century had effectively turned many municipal corporations into electoral colleges, choosing an MP either from among their number or with an eye to protecting the privileges of the corporation. It was this political role in particular which made the corporations prime targets for early-nineteenth-century reformers.[15]

The oligarchies of merchants, prosperous townsmen and sometimes gentry who made up the old corporations were predominantly Anglican Tories. Entry to this elite could be by economic success, although it was commonly perpetuated by co-option according to family status, marriage or the benefits of inheritance. Exclusion by political or religious tests had long been synonymous with corruption in radical circles; by the 1830s it had become a tenet of wider Liberal belief. It was control of the polity and attendant patronage which mattered more than the exercise of any duties. Democracy was to be the new order, ensuring wider participation and a greater openness and accountability to those who paid for the services provided. Councillors elected by the ratepayers and aldermen elected by the councillors would henceforth conduct local government. Separate benches of borough magistrates were also envisaged which would remove judicial functions from administrative authorities. Conveniently, these high-principled reforms were all at the expense of bastions of political conservatism and effectively just handed over control of many town halls to dissenters, radicals and their lower-middle-class supporters. In Reading, for example, reform candidates won fifteen of the eighteen seats up for election after the 1835 Act; only two of the twenty-two members of the old corporation were elected to the new city council.[16] In Leeds only six of the sixty-four councillors and aldermen holding office after those elections had been members of the old corporation.[17] The message was not lost on the Whig hierarchy at Westminster. Lord Ebrington, active in Poor Law reform and matters of public health improvement, wrote enthusiastically to Russell, as Home Secretary, in 1836 that 'the result of the late municipal elections must have convinced the Tories that we have all the most intelligent of the middle class on our side'. With the towns now securely in Liberal hands, and likely to remain so, he calculated that it would be almost impossible for the Tories to govern Britain again.[18]

Whereas Reading, Liverpool, Bristol, Leeds, King's Lynn and Nottingham were all corporations legislated for in the 1835 Act, Bradford, Bolton, Manchester, Birmingham and Sheffield were not. To be able to explain the difference was to understand the mosaic of local government in mid-nineteenth-century Britain. The latter also enjoyed urban self-government, which provided a similar range of functions within prescribed boundaries. They, however, were enabled to do so not by Royal Charter but by the more modern device of Local Acts of Parliament, many of which dated from the eighteenth century. But even here great diversity existed. Local Acts not only created instruments of town government but were also the means of conferring additional powers on those already in existence. Reading held its Charter from 1542 but by the 1830s much of the Corporation's legal empowerment was in fact derived from Local Acts of 1785 and 1826. Local Acts often bore the title of Improvement Acts since they usually authorised a specific body of men, known as Improvement (or Paving) Commissioners, to raise a rate and to undertake the work of repairing and widening roads, lighting streets, removing sewage and waste materials and ensuring adequate drainage in the town by properly designed gutters.

Improvement Commissioners might also have conferred upon them the power of policing, compulsory purchase, building reservoirs for a regular and healthy water supply, and occasionally even setting up a gas works, as in Manchester in 1817. Between 1800 and 1830 alone about 300 such Improvement Commissions were created in British towns and cities.[19] Frequently their functions overlapped with the statutory authority enjoyed by the corporation or even with that which resided at parish or vestry level, the more so when the geographical area of the corporation's or Commissioners' responsibilities encompassed several parishes. But if the responsibilities overlapped, so too – inevitably in local communities – did the personnel. Before 1835 corporation members and Commissioners were frequently the same men wearing different hats – indeed the 1826 Local Act for Reading stipulated that the mayor and Corporation, clergy and county Justices who resided in the borough should all be Improvement Commissioners. Beyond that, 197 other individuals were named.[20] Therein, of course, lay a further question. Even among the restricted numbers who were entitled to participate in early-nineteenth-century local government, how many actively did so and for what reasons other than furthering or defending their vested interests as owners of property, men of business, holders of office or a combination of all? The answer, usually, was very few.

Towns not listed in the schedule of the 1835 Act could none the less benefit from its provisions by a process of incorporation. This might occur if a petition showed convincingly that most inhabitants, including a good proportion of those with wealth and property, desired a new Charter which would legitimise elected councils. This was not, however, a quick or easy procedure. Political opinion was often fiercely divided and counter-petitions and legal challenges could make reform an expensive business for its promoters. No major town beyond those originally listed was incorporated until 1838, when Manchester and Birmingham adopted the new style of elected councils. Nor did the pace of change much quicken thereafter: only fifteen petitions for voluntary incorporation were received by the Privy Council before 1845 and eight of those were rejected.[21] By 1879 the number of municipal boroughs governed under the terms of the 1835 Act was 240 – only sixty-two more than the 178 originally provided for. But that figure disguised broader social change. The 178 corporations of the 1835 schedule contained fewer than 250,000 inhabitants, whereas the 240 boroughs in 1879 had a combined population of over 8 million.[22] Greater numbers, however, did not necessarily mean greater participation or obviously extended benefit. The franchise was restricted to ratepayers of more than two years' standing and until 1869 was often smaller than that for parliamentary elections. In Birmingham, for example, only 3 per cent of the population could vote in the city's elections as late as 1861.[23] A complex system of rateable values also limited those eligible, while plural voting favoured those with property in more than one location. Constraints on eligibility to serve as councillors were even greater. Owning property worth £1,000 or occupying that with a rateable value of £30 per annum in a large borough (£500 and £15 per annum respectively in a small borough) prevented most from ever aspiring to elected office. In any case, service was unpaid and council meetings were held during working hours. Most councillors were shopkeepers, merchants, builders, estate agents, farmers or lawyers. Most shared with their electors the prevailing view that low rates were an indication of efficient and honest administration. Pressure for extensive drainage and sewerage projects or for broadening the remit of councils in any way which meant additional expenditure was unlikely to come from those who would have to pay for it.

Vigilant as ratepayers invariably were, until the last quarter of the nineteenth century the responsibilities of elected authorities remained sufficiently curtailed that apprehensions about reckless spending inspired by vague notions of public betterment were seldom justified. Only after 1880 did the functions of local government come to embrace education, transport, housing and the supply of gas and electricity. The 1835 Act stipulated only one essential duty for the new-style urban authorities: they were obliged to provide a police force to replace the watchmen organised by Improvement Commissioners, which would inevitably be by far the largest item of expenditure. Whether any other responsibilities changed hands depended usually on local will and circumstances. The old corporations were not automatically abolished and the work of Improvement Commissioners in many cases simply continued as before – it too being specified in Acts of Parliament. Before 1845 only in two boroughs, Newcastle-upon-Tyne and Manchester, had the powers of Improvement Commissioners been transferred to the new urban authority.[24] Although the Municipal Corporations Act did expose local government to greater public scrutiny than before, the fact that so many of the new men elected after 1835 were more interested in partisan rivalry than in administrative effectiveness blunted the advantage which might otherwise have accrued from this new democracy. In the 1830s and 1840s manipulating ward boundaries for electoral gain, passing resolutions and forwarding petitions on matters of national importance to London preoccupied many local politicians. The state of the town's roads, gutters and sewers and the removal of hazards to public health were far less exciting and often could conveniently be left to those bodies which had long supervised such mundane matters.

Not only did pre-1835 structures of authority therefore survive but even after that date Local Acts of Parliament continued to be passed in order to confer wider responsibilities upon them. It was a Local Act of 1842, for instance, which transformed the functions of government in Leeds by enhancing the power of the Improvement Commissioners. This Act not only increased their authority in the traditional areas of paving, drainage and street lighting and improvements but then added powers to build public conveniences, erect clocks, build a town hall, suppress vice, control nuisances, ensure minimum housing standards and even to prevent the sale of unfit foodstuffs. The authorities in Liverpool received a similarly pioneering remit by a Local Act in the same year. It was also a Local Act in 1851, and not its incorporation in 1838, which transformed the structure and powers of government in Birmingham. The piecemeal nature of these changes was not perhaps surprising. Since the geography of urban areas varied considerably, so the requirements for legislation varied too. Leeds, from its Royal Charter in 1626, covered thirty-two square miles and its boundaries coincided with those of the medieval parish. Even in 1835 some wards remained sparsely populated and wholly agricultural. The borough of Birmingham was less than half that size. The boundaries of other corporations or Paving Commissions, as in Bradford by 1840, included little more than city centres.[25] Disparities of character and size, overlapping legal responsibilities, conflicts between old and new administrative structures and the willingness or otherwise of dignitaries to seek enhanced powers either by incorporation or by Local Acts all contributed to make each local authority not only unique but usually proud to be so.

Even when greater powers were requested and awarded by Parliament there was no obligation to use them. Divisions in local politics often reflected those at national level and fiercely divided councils were always prone to paralysis. Plans to undertake modern drainage schemes in Leeds fell foul of just such wrangling between 1842 and 1849. In any case, educational provision was the big issue in Leeds at that time, diverting attention from other matters and even splitting the controlling Liberal group. It was also much easier for corporations or Improvement Commissioners to levy rates than to collect them. Undertaking public works projects or buying utility companies, however desirable, might also involve heavy borrowing on unfavourable terms to which a legal challenge could be made. In the 1830s and 1840s many authorities were unsure of the precise limits of their statutory powers; there was little central direction or inspection of their activities. And even where corporation, parish and Commissioners all shared perceptions of the common good, the prospect of commitment to long-term, potentially ruinous and complicated engineering works was daunting for men who lacked professional and scientific training and who had no experience in handling experts unfurling grand architectural plans before them.

Finally, vested interests always resisted both the passing and enforcement of regulations which hindered trade. Chadwick acknowledged this in 1844 when observing that despite specific legislation little had been done to remove the cellar tenements in which many of the urban poor dwelt. This was because so many town councillors were 'largely connected with the small owners or directly interested in that description of property'. Again in 1848 he remarked that he knew of places where two or three manufacturers who dominated the ratepayers prevented any application of the law.[26] Builders were adept at cutting corners whatever standards might be required. Many manufacturers were not only the stalwarts of civic government but also the worst polluters of the environment. If local government in mid-nineteenth-century Britain had one uniform feature it was that it was truly local and overwhelmingly wished to stay so, whatever divisions within its ranks there might be. The age of unitary administrations supervised from London while exercising wide responsibilities for the benefit of their communities as a whole lay far in the future.

To complicate matters further, the important issue of poor relief did not fall within the remit of local government as the 1835 Act defined it. The Whig ministry's measure to tackle rising levels of pauperism in fact predated its reform of the municipal corporations: in 1834 it passed the Poor Law Amendment Act. Like most reform in the 1830s this was a contentious piece of legislation, pitting high ideals and economic theory against the grinding reality of poverty for a large section of the population with whom legislators were unlikely to have much immediate contact. There had always been relief for the destitute and few argued that it should cease. But the conviction, certainly in Liberal circles, was that the old system was breaking down. Welfare provision had to be more efficient and made less attractive to those who were physically able to work. Support for the unemployed maintained wages at artificially high levels by lessening the competition for labour. Charity had its place, but as a moral virtue on the part of those who dispensed it and not as a challenge to natural economic laws.[27]

Relief for paupers had been regulated since the 1590s. The Elizabethan Poor Law, however, had been designed for a predominantly agricultural country with about 4 million inhabitants. By 1834 Britain's economy was industrialising, its population stood at 25 million and its rapidly expanding cities witnessed poverty both on a scale and more concentrated than previously imaginable. Rural underemployment from the 1780s onwards and then economic depression after the Napoleonic Wars had led to unprecedented demands for welfare, well beyond the needs of the aged, sick and abandoned women with children for whom compassion might most readily be justified. By 1815 expenditure on relief in England and Wales had trebled from the estimated level of £2 million in 1784.[28] Responsibility for the poor had always lain with Britain's 15,600 parishes. These were not uniform in size or population: while fifty-four had fewer than ten inhabitants, at the other extreme ten had populations above 50,000.[29] Nevertheless, in each of them a poor rate was collected and an overseer employed with authority to remove anyone likely to become a burden. Allowances might be made to subsidise scant wages or else employment might be offered, usually by farmers, within the parish. For those demonstrably unfit for work relief might be provided indoors by means of accommodation in a workhouse. These were constructed after 1722 and by 1776 around 2,000 had been completed, each providing places for between twenty and fifty inmates. But building and managing a workhouse was not cheap and whenever possible most parishes preferred to make regular payments by way of outdoor relief at only a quarter of the cost. Some even engaged a doctor to tend not only those in the workhouse but also the poor kept in their own homes.

Just as the Municipal Corporations Act followed a Royal Commission, so the new Poor Law was devised after the Royal Commission set up to investigate the need for reform reported in 1834. With Chadwick as one of its authors, the conclusion that a radical revision was needed was almost inevitable. Twenty-six Assistant Commissioners studied different regions, visiting a fifth of all parishes and gathering information from others. The report identified outdoor relief for the able-bodied as the culprit since this distorted the purpose of any Poor Law by confusing mere poverty with outright destitution. Outdoor relief was thus to be abolished and a willingness to enter the forbidding workhouse environment was to be a self-operating test of eligibility. To ease the burden of expense in erecting more of these institutions, parishes would be grouped together into Unions whereby building and management costs could be spread. The Union with its salaried officers thereby became the administrative unit for the new Poor Law. There would be 600 of them in England and Wales.

A large parish might be designated a Union in its own right; for most, though, new boundaries within which to levy the poor rate and to take responsibility for the deserving poor had to be drawn. This was often hastily done and Union boundaries sometimes cut across historic demarcations of counties and boroughs. Bristol provided a chaotic example of this, as one frustrated inspector complained to Chadwick in 1848. Part of the town was governed by the provisions of a Local Act, part was in the Clifton Union and part was in the Bedminster Union. Yet Bristol also had a mayor and Corporation. 'Who are the authorities in such a case?' Chadwick was asked. 'Who are responsible for carrying out your regulations, and *to whom* am I to apply and urge forward in the good work?'[30] Local anomalies notwithstanding, the work of parish Unions was, for the first time, to come under central government supervision by the creation of the Poor Law Commission, renamed the Poor Law Board in 1847. But such checks from Somerset House amounted to little more than ruling in matters referred there and ensuring that the Union and its officers operated within legal limits. As with local government reform, the new Poor Law was intended to give local people powers to regulate their society. Again, as with local government, the people would not have wished it otherwise.

The eyes and ears of the Poor Law Board were the travelling inspectors, each of whom reported on the operations of about thirty Unions within sixteen geographical regions in England and Wales. In 1838 the expenditure of each district averaged £430,000, giving a total annual expenditure of almost £5.5 million. The culture in Somerset House was one of frugality. Aware of the political danger of being thought to be profligate with public money, Chadwick advised Russell, still Home Secretary in 1838, that the number of inspectors, although small, should not be increased and that those members of the government who sought appointments for their protégés should be politely informed that, even within the existing structure of inspection, officers were available for detachment to Ireland now that the provisions of the new Poor Law were being extended there. By his plan for so doing, Chadwick boasted, could 'the existing expenses which excite much outcry be reduced about twelve thousand pounds'.[31] In 1847 the thirty-eight clerks who served the Commissioners petitioned against the miserable remuneration paid to them when contrasted with that paid to staff at the Admiralty, the Board of Ordnance, the War Office, the Paymaster General's Office and the Commission of Woods, Forests and Land Revenue. In all three grades of clerkship those employed at the Poor Law Commission received an average of about 40 per cent less.[32]

In July 1849 the Secretary to the Poor Law Board, Lord Ebrington, reminded its inspectors that travelling costs needed to be kept down with public transport used whenever possible. The inspectors, in turn, were always on the lookout for inappropriate expenditure and any overly generous provision for workhouse inmates. One complained in 1850 that 'I have Unions in which the dietary is very high and expensive, and where from time to time I have called the attention of the Guardians to the matter.'[33] Persuading Guardians of anything, however, was no easy matter. Union Guardians were elected by each parish in numbers proportionate to its size and from among those who paid the poor rate, and it was upon them, acting as a Board, that Parliament bestowed authority to appoint the workhouse manager, the matron, the overseer, the clerk and any other officers whom they thought fit. The elected Guardians, like town councillors in the new corporations, represented both local democracy and local autonomy in motion. As usual there was a considerable overlap in personnel. Boards of Guardians comprised the same civic dignitaries, magistrates, farmers, clergy, professional men and property owners, many with plural voting, as were eligible for town Council elections or who were Improvement Commissioners. As always, it was those who were active who determined how authority was exercised. Attendance by Guardians at Board meetings was about 50 per cent in urban Unions while as low as 30 per cent among those in rural areas.[34] Elections were often uncontested.

Reining in the generosity of Guardians was not the norm; indeed the inspectors' principal task was to ensure that Guardians fulfilled the duties imposed in 1834 as interpreted by the Poor Law Board. Inspectors, however, were thin on the ground and increasingly so since their number was reduced from twenty-one in 1837 to twelve in 1841 and to only nine in 1847.[35] Their districts were enlarged accordingly and many rural Unions received infrequent and perfunctory visits. In any case, the Poor Law Board had few powers of compulsion and its inspectors rarely could do more than cajole and advise. The Board, for instance, might require Unions to alter or extend an existing workhouse but it could not insist that a new one be erected. Nevertheless, model designs were distributed from Somerset House and by 1840 about 350 workhouses had been constructed in Unions where none had previously existed.[36] This was a measure of the co-operation established between inspectors and Guardians in most regions. Though they varied, workhouses generally provided reasonable accommodation, diet and disciplinary regimes and were not the brutal instruments for physically oppressing the poor which contemporary opinion, largely in the north of England, and the writings of Charles Dickens embedded in the popular imagination. After 1834 the workhouse usually contracted both a medical officer and a teacher for its children. As an alternative for some, the Act sanctioned grants for emigration to the colonies; by 1837 about 6,500 persons had been assisted in this way. [37]

Furthermore, outdoor relief did not cease after 1834 as Parliament had intended and as the Poor Law Commissioners tried to enforce. Even where the Guardians were compliant, overseers might still disregard their rulings. At Newark in 1836 money was even diverted from the highway rate in order to circumvent the prohibition on outdoor relief to able-bodied workmen.[38] Helping paupers in their own homes remained the only practical mode of welfare for most Unions, was well established by regional custom and might even be a statement of autonomy by the Guardians against central direction – especially when it was proven to be cheaper than enlarging the workhouse and employing more officers. Putting the able-bodied into workhouses also had the disadvantage that it removed them from the chance of casual labour, thereby depriving farmers in particular of a pool of needy and low-paid workers living close by. Inspectors learned that it was often best to turn a blind eye to the way in which the Poor Law operated at the grassroots and to report to Chadwick and his colleagues in London what they knew the latter wished to hear. With limited sanction and with many Unions to cover, the inspectors in any case had no chance of really understanding the networks of nepotism and supply contracting which commonly existed or the economies made to keep down the poor rate which were hidden from their view. Pushing the wishes of the Poor Law Board upon reluctant Guardians, as one inspector warned in 1850, 'would not only create unpopularity but would also defeat in many cases its own object'.[39]

Left to the whims of Guardians the 1834 Poor Law was, by one measure, fairly successful. Between 1834 and 1840 relief expenditure in England and Wales was reduced by 28 per cent; thereafter, however, the hungry forties soon began to push the level upwards again. In 1843 above 1.3 million individuals (including children) were receiving outdoor relief alone, with half the 600,000 adults classified as able-bodied. By 1848 it was estimated that 2.25 million people or 14 per cent of the population were unemployed, with 1.87 million claiming poor relief.[40] Poor rates, of course, rose accordingly: total relief expenditure increased from £3.7 million in 1840 to almost £4.4 million in 1847.[41] Other factors also make the success of the new system difficult to judge. Tensions always arose where the incidence of pauperism and the poor rate were not uniform across a multi-parish Union and when, therefore, some ratepayers believed that they were subsidising others.

The same was true when levying a poor rate was restricted by legislation; parishes which logic dictated should be amalgamated with the towns they adjoined were sometimes kept in rural Unions because the Local Act which regulated urban government also stipulated a common rate within the corporation's boundaries. Bristol and Exeter were particular examples of this anomaly: the Poor Law inspector wrote despairingly in 1848 that 'nothing short of a repeal of the Local Acts would effect the alterations and changes which a fair measure of justice to all would require'.[42]

The most widespread problem which the Poor Law encountered, however, was that of entitlement to relief by settlement. In theory all paupers belonged to a parish, usually by birth, parentage or marriage, although even before 1834 other grounds for settlement had been introduced. That the parish was the unit for poor relief had been natural in a rural economy with static population, but well before the 1830s migration had made the shortcomings of the parish system obvious. The 1834 Act, however, did not reflect this reality. The individual parish continued to be the legal unit for rating and settlement until 1865, which often led to disparities and disputes even within the same Union. Throughout the 1840s Justices of the Peace in England and Wales issued an average of about 10,000 removal orders, which in each of the peak years of 1840, 1847 and 1849 affected up to 40,000 persons or about 4 per cent of the national total in receipt of relief.[43] In the 1840s this system was widely felt to favour the towns. The towns gained from the years of labour which a migrant might contribute to their prosperity, yet in adversity or old age the migrant had no claim upon the town's charity. Responsibility for welfare, even after years of absence, still rested with the rural parish from which the individual had originally come and to which, as the place of legal settlement, the hapless or aged pauper should therefore be removed.

There were ways around this anachronism. It was often cheaper to give relief than to begin expensive searches and legal proceedings with a view to removal. Where liability was established Unions might also enter into reciprocal arrangements whereby they transferred the cost of relief without needing to move and house the recipient. The Poor Removal Act of 1846 addressed the complex issue of settlement by introducing a five-year residence qualification for relief in any parish. At this point, however, chaos took over. 'The difficulty of ascertaining who is, and who is not, removable is so great as to induce each parish to cast the onus of proving the removability of each pauper upon the parish in which such pauper may be resident for the time being,' one inspector reported in 1847.[44] The Act had intended five years beginning in or after 1846, but in 1849 a legal ruling permitted any period before 1846 to be included. Rural Unions now judged themselves exempted from old obligations arising from settlement and refused support to any pauper not resident within one of their parishes. With power of removal apparently abolished, towns and cities faced a full and immediate responsibility for anyone claiming relief within their boundaries. Leeds faced a sudden increase of up to £4,000 and Norwich and Bradford of close to £5,000 in their annual expenditure on paupers. In Leicester the poor rate immediately doubled.[45]

In Plymouth the poor rate had to be raised by a total of £1,600 annually merely to cover the cost of providing for the poor who had hitherto been paid for by income from other parishes. Then another ruling in the Court of Queen's Bench pronounced this withdrawal by rural Unions to have been illegal and not in any circumstances permissible when individuals were in receipt of welfare according to prior and lawful arrangements. But the damage was done. 'It has done irreparable evil,' the press in Plymouth complained: 'the rural parishes have shifted their burdens very easily!' Much had been written about the drag of the poor in agricultural areas, the paper continued, but there was a conspicuous absence of criticism about the way in which so large a portion of the poor rate levied on the land had been surreptitiously transferred 'to be a charge on the property – lands, houses, factories and other buildings in the towns'.[46] Town and country were locked in an age-old conflict, the Secretary to the Poor Law Board observed in 1850; so long as settlement and removal existed they would bedevil relations between urban and rural Unions and between differing parishes. Chadwick had expressed similar sentiments years earlier. Society had changed and in his opinion those eligible for relief should simply receive it wherever they lived at the time of application.[47] It was a simple but unimplementable idea. The parish structure had many defenders in Parliament and the alternative, it was widely feared, would be a more centrally controlled system. To acknowledge the problem, nevertheless, Parliament reduced the residence qualification to three years in 1861 and to one year in 1865.

It was into this world of fiercely autonomous local authority structures and the parochial antagonisms of a highly fragmented welfare system, all controlled by men whose immediate interests usually dictated as little enterprise as possible, that reformers tried to introduce their vision of central agencies implementing generic legislation. Chadwick and his associates in London were under no illusions. Not only was local hostility acknowledged to be a persistent obstacle, but sometimes it was even difficult to gather information. When the Poor Law Board surveyed 14,414 parishes in England and Wales in 1851, for instance, only 7,892 overseers of relief bothered to reply. Overseers were not employed by the Board, its President, M. T. Baines, reminded the Prime Minister. Consequently, 'the powers of the Board in dealing with any case of remissness or negligence on the part of the overseers are necessarily very limited'.[48] Therein, of course, lay the contradiction within so much of the permissive legislation of the mid-nineteenth century.

The Public Health Act of 1848 was no exception to that contradiction. Like the Municipal Corporations Act and the Poor Law Amendment Act, it prescribed administrative structures but invested them with few powers with which to perform their range of duties. On paper, the Act was a major victory for health campaigners and the General Board of Health which it created marked a new beginning in the state's responsibility for the living conditions of most people. It authorised the formation of local Boards of Health which might regulate sewers, drains, slaughterhouses and offensive trades. The Act conferred upon these Boards the right to remove public health nuisances, to restrict the use of damp cellars for human habitation, to purchase land for parks, burial grounds and public baths, and even to take over private water companies if the owners agreed. They could administer lighting and paving, appoint medical health officers and then levy a rate and borrow money to cover expenditures. In fact, the Public Health Act offered many authorities the opportunity to assume legal powers which could otherwise have been acquired only at considerable expense by new Local Acts. By operating under the guidance of the General Board, local Boards might also have free access to the expert advice of the former's inspectors. Needless to say, bringing such a raft of powers under the supervision of an organ of central government was anathema to all those who had, and who still opposed the Act. For them, Chadwick's vision evoked the nightmare of a socialistic dictatorship riddled with jobbery and all justified under the guise of promoting a public service.

In the face of such resistance perhaps it was understandable that the 1848 Act lacked compulsion: there was no obligation for any local government authority or Board of Guardians to set up a Board of Health. The only circumstances in which the General Board of Health could force a local Board into being was when the death rate, as averaged across the population of an administrative district, exceeded twenty-three per thousand or when at least 10 per cent of the poor rate payers petitioned the General Board for such a body. A death rate of twenty-three per thousand was a stiff test, since even a high mortality rate in the worst slum areas was unlikely sufficiently to raise the average across a whole town or parish Union. A petition at least acknowledged the principle of local initiative and on receipt of one the General Board would send inspectors to investigate. But an enquiry would then need to be satisfied that a gerrymandering minority was not imposing itself upon the community at large and that the petitioners included in their number an adequate representation of respectable opinion and property ownership. To lobby for a Board of Health usually widened political divisions in any borough or Union and might lead to recriminations lasting years. Radicals and reformers perceived them as instruments of social progress, heedless that they might amount to little more than magistrates, councillors, Improvement Commissioners and Guardians acting under another name. As with so much mid-nineteenth-century change, symbolic triumph was often a greater touchstone of success than functional reality.

Even so, by December 1848 twenty-five towns had applied for the provisions of the 1848 Public Health Act to be adopted either by petitions from ratepayers or from the town Council. Most prominent among these were York, Derby, Wolverhampton, Dover, Portsmouth, Gloucester, Worcester, Preston and Leicester. Chadwick, of course, was delighted, exclaiming at once that 'this body of applications puts an end to the talk of universal resistance'.[49] He was, however, premature. Even boroughs mindful of the need to improve their record on public health did not always look to the 1848 legislation as a model. Local Acts could still best suit specific needs and especially when, after 1847, the cost of securing parliamentary legislation was much reduced by the Clauses

Act, which introduced a procedure for simply transferring standardised legal provisions from one Bill to another. Birmingham, Leeds and Bradford all declined to adopt the 1848 Act and obtained greater powers by means of Improvement Acts instead.[50] Another difficulty with the 1848 Act was that the General Board of Health might require changes to the boundaries of a local Board which made them different from those of the local government authority. Clashes of interest and political rivalry, as in Reading, might then paralyse the local Board as a mechanism for improvement.[51] Persistent inactivity and non-attendance made members liable to disqualification, but where a Board came to be dominated by those unsympathetic, as at Sheerness, it could thereby effectively vote itself out of existence.[52] Central control was essential if such behaviour was to be prevented, Carlisle acknowledged, 'when the local Boards are elected by the ratepayers and may consist of we know not whom'.[53] But in these circumstances the General Board of Health, in reality, could do next to nothing. After three years in post, Carlisle was well acquainted with both the General Board's unpopularity and its limited effectiveness. Advising the Prime Minister on the need for a London Health Bill in 1849, he suggested that the General Board need have no more than a consultative role. It was better to confront reality and 'to have recourse as much as possible to existing bodies, the Boards of Guardians, and the Select Vestries', he concluded, 'putting under them the paving and ordinary sewage works'.[54]

In addition to its modest remit the General Board was poorly funded. The Chancellor of the Exchequer, Sir Charles Wood, was a committed free-trader with no enthusiasm for increased expenditure in order to expand the role of central government in society. At the outset the Board's staff at Gwydyr House in Whitehall was too small for its workload and by 1850 its Secretary, Henry Austin, was so exhausted that he resigned to become a superintending inspector instead. Only two medical inspectors, Richard Grainger and John Sutherland, were appointed to cover England, Wales and Scotland. These men, predictably, were almost entirely dependent upon the co-operation of the Boards of Guardians or town councils with whom they had to deal. Furthermore, it was sometimes unclear whether a proper Board of Health existed in the vicinity. Chadwick complained of the arrangements made at Sunderland in 1848 as apparently lacking any sanction from the Poor Law Guardians. 'We do not know if we do send down any regulations,' he reflected, 'whether the local Board is so constituted as to execute them.'[55] At every level impediments to tackling the filth and disease of Britain's towns seemed to render legislation useless. Austin observed in 1849 how 'it has been found that there is a very great indisposition among householders to sign papers that are to be made the instrumentality of taking legal proceedings against their neighbours'.[56] Although the 1848 legislation allowed public officials to bring actions for nuisance removals, witnesses were still needed and officers of local Boards of Health had to be initially alerted. House-to-house inspections, when Guardians would pay for them, were unpopular among the poor. It had been assumed by many middle-class reformers that the latter would be pleased to have their insanitary accommodation visited and the incidence of sickness thereby reduced, but the inquisitorial nature of the event invaded the privacy and offended the instincts of even the humblest Englishmen. It would take a lot more than permissive Acts of Parliament to translate the zeal of such men as Chadwick, Southwood-Smith, Slaney, Ashley and Austin into cleaner streets and underground sewers.

Reports from inspectors, evidence to Royal Commissions, and investigations by reformers and local authorities combined to reveal the scale of the problem which had to be confronted. Chadwick calculated that 62 per cent of towns had insufficient or impure water supplies. Most cities stank from overflowing cesspools, dung heaps and horse manure in the summer while in the winter their streets would often be awash with effluence. Cattle were driven into city centres for slaughter: London alone had 1,500 privately owned abattoirs in the mid-nineteenth century which simply discharged blood and offal into notional gutters. Gateshead, with a population of 25,000 in the 1840s, had thirty-one abattoirs. Cowsheds, ill-ventilated and ill-drained, were likewise located in the centres of towns and pig keeping was commonplace among urban people in order to provide cheap meat. Reading, for instance, was estimated to have 378 pigsties in 1847 for its population of 17,000.

London had 3,000 known cesspools in 1841. Leicester had the same number for its 50,000 people. For many of the urban poor, cesspools were the closest thing to sanitation. Having no access to a privy, holes, ditches or a nearby stream would serve their needs and night soil was commonly deposited in alleyways, courtyards and public thoroughfares. There was an agricultural market for dung which meant that some accumulations were eventually transported by contractors, but this was not a realistic solution to the problem where the cost of removal exceeded its saleable value. In any case, guano imports soon became the preferred agricultural fertiliser. As late as the 1840s some sizeable towns still had no sewers. Croydon in 1848 lacked all but the crudest drainage for its 13,000 inhabitants. Hitchin with 7,000 and even Dudley with 40,000 people likewise lacked sewerage systems. Others might boast a sewer, but for no good reason. Winchester's 15,000 inhabitants were not served by the one sewer connected only to the army barracks. The town had one central well and was renowned for its endemic typhoid fever. Reading, one of the places which had a mortality rate higher than twenty-three per thousand in the 1840s, was singled out by Southwood-Smith as a particularly dirty and insanitary town. Its 17,000 inhabitants lived in 4,155 houses, half of which had no water supply. For 95 per cent of the borough there was no drainage; cesspools constantly overflowed into the river and streams. In Finsbury and Holborn only one-third of the houses were linked to the London sewers. When it came to deficient sanitation and its concomitant diseases those who lived and worked in the metropolis were never unaware of the nation's problems.[57]

The task of addressing these problems went well beyond political campaigners, energetic bureaucrats, local reform associations and those magistrates, clergy, councillors and Guardians who took seriously their duties in towns and parishes nationwide. It involved too the expanding class of professional men whose expert evidence and scientific opinion increasingly became the determining factor in overcoming opposition to and then implementing the large-scale projects so desperately needed. Scientific analysts alone could pronounce with authority on the quality of water supply. Architects and engineers were needed not just for conceptual vision but for the building of pumping stations, networks of underground sewers, pipe construction and to determine the appropriate materials to be used in manufacture.[58] Among professionals, however, the group most in daily contact with the dire effects of inadequate public health were medical practitioners, many of whom were themselves active in national and local campaigns for improvement. Legislation required definitions and then judgments which in the eyes of the Law could be given only by those formally qualified. Who could identify a health hazard? Who could say whether a nuisance had been the cause of illness or death? A profession held low in public esteem at the beginning of the nineteenth century by the 1840s found itself elevated as a source of scientific truth and a promoter of social progress.[59]

It was not always easy to justify that elevation. Revelations about Burke and Hare in 1828 became a national sensation and even in the early 1830s grave robbers plying their trade to satisfy the demand from anatomy schools were still being apprehended. Nepotism, corruption and malpractice exposed among physicians in the 1820s also became public scandals; the common perception of medical men was as grasping and incompetent – not perhaps surprising in a profession so loosely regulated. In theory the medical world comprised three separate callings of physicians, surgeons and apothecaries. Physicians were predominantly graduates from the ancient or Scottish universities who diagnosed and advised for those who could afford to consult them. Physicians aspired to be gentlemen. They did not cut flesh nor, if avoidable, lay hands upon a patient. Within seven miles of London numbers were limited by the need for a licence from the Royal College of Physicians, founded in 1518, but in provincial towns practice was determined by the market for their services. Most of Britain's thousand or more physicians in the 1840s made a good and sometimes handsome living and their social status distinguished them from the nation's remaining 16,000 medical practitioners who were categorised as surgeons.

Surgeons were represented by their own Royal College, established in 1800, which distanced them from an ancient association with barbers. They were expected to undergo a five-year apprenticeship followed by courses and clinical experience in a recognised hospital in London, Edinburgh, Glasgow or Dublin. This branch of the profession grew rapidly in the early nineteenth century. When founded, the Royal College of Surgeons had a thousand members; by 1850 more than 8,000 were registered. An enormous expansion in medical education took place in private medical schools both in London and across the country, facilitated by the Anatomy Act of 1832, which abolished many of the previous restrictions on dissection. By the 1840s these private schools had either disappeared or been amalgamated and medical training was becoming focused on the four major hospitals of Guy's,

St Bartholemew's, St Thomas's and the London Hospital. A more identifiable structure of education helped to raise the surgeons' status and by the 1840s a hospital senior surgeon might enjoy the standing once reserved for successful physicians.[60] Association with government enquiries or with regulatory bodies might raise his status yet further.

The third estate of medicine, apothecaries, had been regulated by their Worshipful Society since 1617 and more recently by the Apothecaries Act of 1815. They were licensed after a five-year apprenticeship which involved attending lectures and hospital practice and examination on their knowledge of the drugs and concoctions which physicians and surgeons might require. Technically, apothecaries were tradesmen whose livelihood was derived from selling their wares. Many kept their own shops while others were supplied from the shops of druggists. But apothecaries had a dual function. While they were obliged to provide what more exalted professionals prescribed they were also the first call for many among the poor who needed help and they might visit and treat patients in their own homes while selling medicines. In country areas surgeons often supplied their own prescriptions and might style themselves surgeon-apothecaries. By the early nineteenth century, however, that was not the only way in which the traditional tripartite division had effectively broken down.

Unqualified medical practice was not illegal until the Medical Act of 1858, when it was discovered, as the public had long suspected, that only one-third of all practitioners had a diploma of any sort.[61] Quackery thrived amid the gullible poor, where expense or a fear of savage surgical procedures might make more conventional attention a last resort. Not all such providers, however, were intent on fraud. The Reverend John Guyther in rural Yorkshire had no medical education, yet in the 1830s and 1840s he issued medicines regularly to his parishioners and was invariably called to their bedsides.[62] But even among those properly qualified in the early nineteenth century the changing nature of medical practice had given rise to a new type of professional – the general practitioner. Indeed, by the 1840s a minority of medical men were exclusively physicians or surgeons and most were applying their skills and knowledge according to the criterion of patient demand. Overcrowding within the profession, which all complained of, contributed further to the erosion of old demarcations. By the 1840s Britain's authorities licensed between 800 and a thousand new doctors every year when to preserve an overall ratio of one to 1,100 heads of population, and thereby a reasonable level of remuneration, required an annual recruitment of merely five hundred.[63]

It was ironic then that an age characterised by increasing competition for work and concomitant hardship for many young men struggling to establish an adequate clientele should also see a rising profile for the profession, at least among the liberal intelligentsia, as an agent for necessary reforms. The Poor Law Amendment Act gave official recognition to the place of doctors when requiring that each Union should make provision for those on relief and in the workhouses. General Medical Orders of the Poor Law Board in 1842 issued standard guidance for parish surgeons and provided for the division of the 600 or so Unions in England and Wales into about 2,800 medical districts, each of which should have a resident medical officer tending no more than a population of 15,000 or an area of 15,000 acres.[64] But implementation was patchy and the terms and conditions of employment were hardly generous – nor did those who framed the new Poor Law intend that they should be. A system of tendering after public advertisement was designed to drive down the medical budgets of all parish Unions and if local men would not do the job for near-subsistence pay then unemployed graduates from London or Edinburgh would be sought who would be grateful for the opportunity. 'Surely *wholesale* medical attendance ought to be cheaper than *retail*,' Chadwick was advised by one of his inspectors in 1836, 'and I expect to *save* upon the present medical contracts which are by *single parishes* whereas under the new system they are to be by *wholesale districts*.'[65] Many medical districts were in fact a good deal larger than the 1842 Orders allowed: two Union surgeons shared Leeds's 88,000 inhabitants. for example, while six in Liverpool had catchment populations of 37,000 apiece. Manchester had five Union surgeons for a population of 160,000. Hull had only one for 41,000 inhabitants. Annual medical costs came to only £150,000 in the mid-1840s at a time when the total expenditure on poor relief in England and Wales topped £4.5 million[66] – not perhaps surprising when some young surgeons were obliged to take part-time Union work for as little as £20 per annum and with no security of tenure. Their willingness to do so was held to demonstrate good character, professional zeal and a commitment to the wider community which in time would be rewarded by the patronage of those who could afford to pay them properly. The surgeons of the Halifax Union felt such despair that in 1849 they submitted a petition to Parliament pointing out the great disparity of pay between those who cared for the poor and those engaged by the Army, the police and even the prison service.[67]

Not all their colleagues were quite so desperate. Within the framework of the Poor Law and the new legislation in the field of public health there were increasing opportunities for crusading doctors to impress upon both the public and divisional magistrates the contribution they could make to a better society. The 1846 Nuisances Act, for instance, allowed a local government authority to take legal action against the owners of health hazards on the recommendation of two qualified medical men, thereby relieving, at least to some extent, the burden of prosecution from the occupiers of adjacent property and making medical judgement the test of the law. The Act went further towards recognising the value of professional expertise by allowing Boards of Health, where they existed, to appoint medical officers to operate within their areas of jurisdiction. Leicester in 1846, Liverpool in 1847 and London in 1848 made such appointments and a further four towns did so by 1866. But Local Acts still mattered. Both William Duncan in Liverpool and John Simon in the City of London were appointed according to the provisions of specific Improvement Acts.[68]

Within the Poor Law structure not all surgeons fared badly. The poor among Exeter's 31,000 population were well served by four Union surgeons. The larger London Unions generally employed enough practitioners: Stepney had five who together treated about 8,000 patients every year and, as elsewhere, undertook midwifery and pioneering work in vaccinating against the ravages of smallpox. The average annual stipend for a Union surgeon in Britain was £69 and many could afford to quit such work after a few years as a reputation for good general practice developed. In 1848 65 per cent of the 16,485 practitioners in England and Wales were indeed able to support themselves by private practice alone. But at any time during the 1840s about 20 per cent of medical men worked within the Poor Law system and, given the rapid turnover, a far higher percentage would have experienced such work at some time in their careers.[69]

Parish surgeons travelled distances in all weathers visiting the most squalid habitations and frequently having to meet the costs of drugs and dressings themselves. When there was widespread illness in the district a surgeon might be mercilessly overworked and requests for temporary assistants were usually declined. Union surgeons operated within a system which, while recognising their growing status as experts, effectively tied their hands at every turn. Relations with employing Guardians were often strained and without any tenure or security the scope for protest against the whims and actions of a local authority was small. Sometimes others spoke on their behalf. A retired physician in Manchester complained to the Poor Law Board in 1849 that 'unpleasant contentions are almost daily arising between the medical men engaged in the service and the Boards of Guardians or other controlling authorities'.[70] This was no doubt true, but few other physicians would have expressed similar sympathy. Sutherland told Chadwick in 1847 of the considerable antipathy which the latter felt towards the humble parish surgeon: 'They are generally considered to be the enemies of the profession who undersell their brethren.'[71]

The General Board of Health sometimes chivied local authorities to lighten the medical officers' load, as when it directed the St Pancras Guardians to take on four extra doctors while cholera raged in London. But the General Board could not insist and the St Pancras Guardians, like others in 1849, simply refused.[72] Power lay with Poor Law Guardians or borough councillors, who rarely wished to employ a man too eager in his part-time duties and whose principal responsibility in any case was to ensure that rates were kept low and that such expenditure as could not be avoided provided the best return. While the Acts of 1834 and 1835 reshaped first the system of poor relief and then the composition of municipal government, the new structures put in place for both remained essentially the domain of those who paid for them and those who were free to give their time to public duties. Cholera would test these different strands of local authority in mid-nineteenth-century Britain to the utmost. Nowhere would that be more so than in the great naval port of Plymouth.

CHAPTER 2

The Boroughs and Unions of South Devon

PLYMOUTH WAS AN ancient borough with a Royal Charter dating from 1440.[1] It returned two members to Parliament and was typical of the old-style municipal corporations reformed by the Act of 1835. The new Town Council which followed consisted of thirty-six Councillors elected from six wards and twelve aldermen. Once in place, the Council created committees to deal with specific duties, chief among which by the late 1840s were the committees of management and the watch, finance, water and land. As elsewhere, Liberals and Tories vied for power although the latter always struggled to throw off the stigma of association with the old oligarchy which had previously run the unreformed Corporation. The *Plymouth and Devonport Weekly Journal*, edited by the radical Isaac Latimer,[2] applauded the revolution which had been effected since 1835 and missed no opportunity to remind its readers that in the era of Tory dominance corruption, extravagance and fraud had been rife within a body comprising pompous men of wealth, high birth but no ability. Whatever upheavals existed in Plymouth politics, however, never seemed to affect the calm disposition of its town clerks: the office was held by only two incumbents in all the years between 1780 and 1879.[3]

The politics of Plymouth were by no means confined to its Council. Like most towns in Britain, the administration was divided between the Corporation, Improvement Commissioners and a Board of Guardians of the poor, all deriving their authority from parliamentary statute. Fundamental to local government were the Improvement Acts of 1770 and 1824. These Acts had conferred powers over paving, lighting, watching and improving the town upon Commissioners drawn from the ranks of those with a personal estate of £2,000 or with property rated above £50 per annum. Commissioners were elected by men with property rated above £20 per annum. By contrast, the qualification for voting in parliamentary elections was only half that figure and in elections for the Town Council all ratepayers were enfranchised. The Municipal Corporations Act had allowed for powers to be transferred to elected councils but no transfer of any responsibilities had occurred in Plymouth. The Commissioners held monthly meetings at the Guildhall, otherwise conducting their business, like the Town Council, via a series of committees covering management, improvement, lighting, rates and finance. After 1835 a special committee was needed whose task was to consult with the Town Council in areas of overlapping jurisdiction.

Inevitably there were tensions between the two: at a heated meeting on 19 September 1849 one Councillor rounded on the dual governance of the town. 'The working of the two bodies, both Commissioners and Town Council, had become entirely a political affair,' he complained. 'The consequence of that was the mal-formation of committees and this resulted in bad management.'[4] But the mayor soon put a stop to the criticism. The fact was that many men were members of both bodies and, in practice, since both Councillors and Commissioners, once elected or co-opted, were likely to remain in office for as long as they wished their interests were not served by such outbursts. Neither Council nor Commission had any real desire to alter the way in which Plymouth was governed, each being content merely to defend and if possible to extend its authority in relation to the other.

By the late 1840s both bodies had sizeable debts and every year they underwent the tortuous exercise of setting and then trying to collect their rates and agonising over the legal limits of their borrowing capacities. In 1852 the Corporation's debt stood at over £52,000.[5] In 1848 the Council spent £1,800 beyond its income, to cover which it issued new bonds to the value of £2,000. Its principal commitment was an £8,000 loan for building a new gaol. For many years the Improvement Commission had tried to keep down its costs by refusing to connect properties to its drains unless an extra payment beyond the normal rate was made. This policy was reversed in 1837, although many in the town complained that it made little difference. Whereas the water supply was controlled by the Council, drains and sewers were undoubtedly the Commissioners' responsibility; in some parts of Plymouth, however, their hands were tied by being unable to insist that new developments should be constructed with any facilities at all.

Other problems were likewise not always their fault. Contractors failed to honour their commitments to remove household refuse, the police did nothing when the law was infringed and workmen blocked the sewers by sweeping in rubble from the streets rather than taking it away. The rate which the Commissioners could levy was also capped – the more so after 1835 when watching duties were relinquished. While capping was much to the relief of many inhabitants, who had a poor opinion of the service provided, it obviously made large-scale projects difficult to plan even when the will existed. The Improvement Commissioners were able to raise £6,354 in 1848, which was manifestly insufficient to meet the projected costs of £7,000 for two schemes in prospect, the ordinary maintenance expenditures of the town and to make provision for the £15,000 of debt which the Commission already carried.[6] Whatever its shortcomings might be, though, the Commission vehemently refuted the accusation that one-third of Plymouth remained effectively undrained.

Like many British cities, Plymouth had experienced rapid growth in the early nineteenth century and some unregulated building on the outskirts of the old town had occurred. Plymouth's population was only 16,000 in 1801. It was 31,000 in 1831, more than 36,000 in 1841 and over 52,000 by the middle of the century. New housing, however, had not remotely kept pace with this increase in numbers and by the 1840s overcrowding was common in districts where larger houses, once of the middle classes, had been abandoned to dangerous levels of multi-occupancy. Whereas the town's population had grown by nearly 34,000 between 1800 and 1850, only about 1,400 new houses had been built and with an average of ten occupants per property Plymouth's density was twice the national average. Nevertheless it was a bustling port with many emigrants passing through it and with sizeable Jewish and Irish communities. Plymouth also served as an important market and traditional manufacturing centre for south Devon and east Cornwall; in particular it was the major cattle market for the region with slaughterhouses and cowsheds familiar features even amid the narrow streets. Vagrancy became a very noticeable problem in the late 1840s as agricultural distress drove many off the land. This was a reason why the Town Council was so ready to incur a greater burden of debt for a larger prison.

Prior to 1914 Plymouth remained administratively distinct from its two neighbours, East Stonehouse and Devonport. By the mid-nineteenth century East Stonehouse was already contiguous with Plymouth, whereas Devonport was still just physically separated. East Stonehouse was a parish: it comprised about a thousand houses and 10,000 inhabitants. Having no Local Act, it was governed by Justices and parish officers, many of whom also sat on an elected Board of Guardians deriving its authority from the Select Vestry Act of 1819. When the provisions of the Poor Law Amendment Act were implemented in 1837 East Stonehouse was created a single-parish Union. The Board of Guardians then became its predominant authority, remaining so until an urban council was created in 1894.

Devonport, known as Plymouth Dock until 1824, was a borough identified by Local Acts of 1781 and 1814 covering both Devonport and the wider parish of Stoke Damerel, of which it was a part. These Acts conferred powers of paving, lighting, nuisance removal and watching on a Board of 160 Improvement Commissioners, many of whom were elected by inhabitants rated at above £8 per annum. The Local Acts also placed responsibility for relieving the poor with these Commissioners, thereby making that body a Board of Guardians. It retained that status even after the 1834 Act, which reorganised Stoke Damerel as a parish Union but did not override the complex provisions of previous Local Acts. Notwithstanding, the Borough was the first in Britain to petition for incorporation after 1835 and in 1836 it thereby acquired a Town Council, with a mayor and the usual annual elections, to which the duty of watching was transferred. Unlike Plymouth, Devonport was a Tory stronghold – much to Latimer's disgust. His paper's bias was never more blatantly displayed than when reporting two Tory losses on the Council in 1849: 'We are glad of this,' the *Journal* trumpeted. The Liberals, it was hoped, would do better still next time.[7]

Separate as the three towns were politically, all made up the large urban centre, three miles across, which had developed around the port of Plymouth and its proximate naval installations. Devonport was popularly perceived as the daughter town of Plymouth. This was a somewhat patronising view given that Stoke Damerel had about 34,000 inhabitants by the mid-1840s, most of whom lived in

Devonport, and that in recognition of its size the Borough had been awarded two parliamentary seats in the redistribution of 1832 although its parliamentary boundaries also took in the voters of East Stonehouse. The Local Act of 1814 none the less had acknowledged Plymouth's standing by stipulating that the mayor, aldermen and Recorder of Plymouth should always be among Devonport's Commissioners. It stipulated too that the Lord of the Manor of East Stonehouse should *ex officio* be included. Forming one urban community, as the three towns effectively did, the state of health of the inhabitants of one was the natural concern of all. In fact when it came to public welfare the integration of Plymouth, East Stonehouse and Devonport was openly acknowledged. Poor relief transcended town boundaries and there was no issue of legal settlement – as was made abundantly plain in 1843 when the assistant overseer of the Stoke Damerel Union surveyed the number of non-resident paupers receiving outdoor relief. 'When I speak of non-resident relief I do not intend to include the neighbouring towns of Plymouth or Stonehouse,' he reported. 'We consider persons residing there as being resident paupers as they are as much under our own inspection as if actually residing in the parish.'[8] The three towns, although in different Poor Law Unions, also had reciprocal arrangements regarding the duties of their parish surgeons. Stoke Damerel employed two surgeons, but one of them could be called upon by the overseers of both Plymouth and East Stonehouse to attend to any sick poor in need.

Although Devonport gained parliamentary representation and a Town Council in the 1830s, the Improvement Commissioners, doubling as the Board of Guardians, still formed its effective instrument of government in the late 1840s. The Commissioners' dual status was deplored by the Poor Law Board in London because of the opportunity it gave for mixing up the accounts, but Local Acts being as they were it was impossible to intervene. By contrast, the authorities in East Stonehouse could not obscure their workings behind any Local Act, since there was none. They did so instead behind entrenched officers who frequently made access to information and auditing as difficult as possible. The Rodd family was a conspicuous part of this network of interest which effectively ran the Union.

Family ties were common features within nineteenth-century local government and in the tight-knit communities of town and parish survived beyond the 1835 reform. They existed not only among the men elected to public office but also among those who served as clerks to the vestries, Councils, Commissioners, magistrates and Guardians. These functionaries were rarely salaried employees; they were predominantly lawyers who treated the authority as a client and who habitually presented inflated bills to cover time and expenses. Many solicitors acted on behalf of different administrative and legal bodies simultaneously and the business was frequently passed from father to son or between partners in the same firm, in some cases through several generations.[9] Richard Rodd's career was therefore not unusual. He became clerk to the Poor Law Guardians of East Stonehouse in 1837. He was clerk to the Justices and also served as solicitor to the parish after 1833. He still held all these positions in 1850. Before he moved to East Stonehouse he had been for eight years solicitor to the parish of Stoke Damerel, where he had also been town clerk, and had helped his father who for years had been solicitor to many parishes in the surrounding area. Together with his father and brother-in-law he had acted as a clerk to other divisional Justices. And to carry on the tradition his son, Robinson Rodd, was engaged by the parish of East Stonehouse in the late 1840s as his assistant. Rodd was accused of making excessive legal charges over many years. Furthermore, the poor rate in East Stonehouse had long been much higher than that levied in either Plymouth or Devonport, yet the accounts of the parish, unlike those of its neighbours, were never published. Rodd refuted all this and gained testimonials as to his upright character from more than seventy local worthies.[10]

The most serious allegations against Rodd, however, related to electoral malpractice. With political rivalry by no means confined to reformed Town Councils, contests for Union and parish authorities could be equally intense and where Liberals and Tories manoeuvred to dominate Boards of Guardians it was common for elections to be challenged by accusations of sharp practice. The scope for fraud was indeed considerable. Guardian elections were very different from the open ballots for parliamentary seats, being conducted instead by means of papers handed out to ratepayers for collection on completion. The system invited irregularities in both distribution and recovery. It allowed too for votes to be altered subsequently or for party agents to fill in forms in advance. Enquiries at Clitheroe and Bolton in 1847, and more extensively at Leeds in 1852, exposed the extent of corruption possible.

But malpractice went further than manipulating democratic procedures. The appointment of overseers, their assistants and other Union officers, though nominally supervised by the Poor Law Board, was frequently determined by local patronage and political intrigue. It was often overseers who kept the register of ratepayers, and hence electors, up to date. Liverpool, Leeds and Salford in the 1840s provided glaring examples of tampering with the register for political advantage, usually by backdating rate payments or neglecting to record them as elections drew near. In Salford there were challenges to two-thirds of the names on the list of electors produced by the overseer.[11]

In East Stonehouse keeping the register was the clerk's job, wearing his hat as Returning Officer, and, according to his critics, Rodd was adept at finding spurious means of disqualifying voters who did not support his preferred candidates. The evidence against him was specific and given greater credibility by the fact that since only about two hundred inhabitants were eligible to vote for the Guardians in East Stonehouse Rodd's ability to disqualify up to sixty voters, as he was reported to have done in 1849, would obviously make such efforts worthwhile. When applications for checking the official book were made it was always mysteriously lost and Rodd's private notes had to be used, among which there were outrageously few references to men newly moved into the parish and about whose politics, presumably, Rodd had as yet discovered nothing.[12] In response, Rodd accused those who whispered against him of acting vindictively. Whatever the details, the authority in East Stonehouse was clearly manipulated by a faction among the Guardians on whose behalf Rodd applied his legal skills. It was a much smaller administrative structure than that of Plymouth and untouched by the reforming provisions of 1835. The Guardians and Justices of East Stonehouse were certainly not accustomed to public scrutiny.

Whereas in East Stonehouse the Board of Guardians was the organ of government, in Plymouth the remit of the Guardians was more focused on tending the poor and running the workhouse. The Plymouth Poor Law Union had been created by uniting the town's two parishes of St Andrew and Charles the Martyr before 1834. By 1849 the former had 2,155 payers of the poor rate, while the latter yielded 1,438. A

Local Act capped at £6,000 the total which the Guardians could raise in a single year and no further rate could be levied until the period for which the former applied had expired. Parliament had envisaged that from time to time circumstances might arise in which more than £6,000 was needed, in which case the Justices in Quarter Sessions could be applied to for legal authority to raise a higher sum. The Municipal Corporations Act transferred this discretionary power to the Plymouth Town Council.

By the late 1840s £6,000 had ceased to be a realistic figure and the Guardians had been forced to borrow money privately from one of their number in advance of future collections. In 1847 an ingenious loophole was devised whereby two rates, amounting to £17,000, were levied during the forthcoming year – legally permissible, the Poor Law Board ruled, as long as they did not run concurrently. But this practice proved unpopular and was abandoned. The Guardians then applied to the Town Council for authority to raise a poor rate of £16,000 in quarterly instalments for the year 1849–50. The application was unanimously approved. Of that total £700 was for debts carried over from previous years. More than £2,000 of income due remained uncollected.

Among the fifty-two Guardians of the Plymouth Union, thirty-eight were directly elected and fourteen were nominated by the Town Council. This appearance of democracy, however, disguised more than just the property qualifications for both electors and elected. One ratepayer described an election for a Guardian in the St Andrew vestry in 1851. The vicar, his clerk, churchwardens and a few others assembled and within a couple of minutes the vicar's clerk was proposed. When the innocent ratepayer suggested another candidate he was brusquely told by a current Guardian who owed his own position to the officers of the vestry: 'You fool, there will be no seconder.'[13] Following the predicted silence the vicar's clerk was duly returned. Attendance at Board meetings was also a problem. An inquorate gathering in 1849 had to wait over an hour before sufficient Guardians could be summoned by messengers in order for business to be conducted. One wag suggested while waiting that 'in future their meetings should be called at the sound of 'fife and drum'– the Guardians might be got to turn out by that means'.[14] In theory absentees could be fined but in practice no fine was ever imposed. In consequence, 'every ratepayer's nerves cannot bear the bullying of some 20 or 30 Guardians', one disgruntled

Guardian observed in 1851.[15] As in East Stonehouse, the routine business of the Board was conducted by an officer of long standing and extensive local knowledge, Robert Burnard, who by 1849 had been clerk to the Plymouth Guardians for over thirty years.

After January 1847 the Poor Law inspector for the West Country, within whose region all the Unions of Cornwall, Devon, Dorset, Gloucester, Somerset and Wiltshire fell, was Edward Gulson. Within four years Gulson had concluded that 'the administration at Plymouth is vicious and unsatisfactory and will so remain till it is placed under some other authority'.[16] At the root of the problem, he believed, were all the Local Acts which bestowed specific privileges and powers upon boroughs such as Plymouth and Devonport, thereby setting them beyond the control of the Poor Law Board in London. Gulson was a conscientious man and not given to hasty judgement; he also had considerable experience of the operation of the new Poor Law, having been an inspector in Ireland between 1838 and 1845, where he had helped to set up the system, and then an inspector in central England and parts of Wales during 1846. His expertise was recognised when he was called to give evidence to a committee of the House of Lords on Irish poor relief in 1849. He was an astute observer of economic conditions and of the management problems of individual workhouses. He also gathered statistical data and took a delight in reading and compiling annual reports. Gulson was a stickler for detail and for efficient administrative procedures, sparing himself no more than he spared others. When he took up new duties in 1846 he requested from the Poor Law Board copies of all orders issued to Boards of Guardians and a set of all reports on English Unions. Confident in his intellectual abilities and knowing both Russell, now Prime Minister, and Chadwick from their work in Poor Law reform over many years, Gulson not only did his job – he believed in it.

The task of approving the accounts of Unions and their workhouses lay not with the Poor Law inspectors but with district auditors who reported directly to Somerset House. This, however, did not deter Gulson from scrutinising the finances of Unions in his region. Boards of Guardians were supposed to complete forms indicating payments for outdoor and indoor relief: Gulson kept copies of all these and then, when he visited, compared the figures against entries in the Union's ledgers. Not resting there, he then added up the returns for each block of twenty-six weeks in order to check the total with the half-yearly abstract which the Union was also required to make up. 'By these comparisons I have from time to time discovered many irregularities and improper alterations of the accounts,' he exclaimed.[17] No one would have doubted it. Coming to Plymouth, East Stonehouse and Devonport in 1847, so thorough an inspector would find rich pickings amid the chaotic way in which these Unions kept their books and managed the workhouses.

Under the provisions of the 1824 Local Act the method by which Guardians of the poor in Plymouth were to keep accounts was not laid down in any detail. The principle by which they should operate, however, was that expenditure in any year should be covered by the rate levied in that year. This was designed to ensure that costs were borne by those responsible for the expenditure and could not become a charge upon the inhabitants of future years, many of whom may not even have been resident at the time. Estimating for a year in advance was never easy, especially since borrowing money commercially was not permitted because the interest owed would constitute a charge carried forward to the following year. The Guardians' practice of collecting the poor rate by instalments was also unlawful, it transpired, since no mention of such a procedure was made in the Local Act. Since concurrent rates were illegal and since the inhabitants would not accept more than one rate to be set per annum, the Guardians always faced the possibility of an annual shortfall. The Poor Law Board urged a system of rates levied for shorter periods at different times during the year, and to be paid immediately, as the only solution. They, of course, did not have the difficult task of collecting the money from the citizens of Plymouth.

But legal restrictions from the past could not explain away all that was wrong with the finances of the Plymouth Guardians. Rate receipt books were improperly kept by some collectors and when Gulson tried to trace what debts were outstanding he found the records useless. The district auditor, William Hughes, had no greater success and received even less co-operation. Describing one occasion when he pointed out to the Guardians that the books for the year were not made up and that the account did not balance, Hughes reported to London that the meeting became 'very noisy and tumultuous' and that 'I found it extremely difficult to preserve sufficient order to carry on the business'.

In the end the attempt to do so had to be abandoned.[18] Even Gulson had never encountered a Union run like this before.

Although it was hard to discover what was buried in their ramshackle accounting system, the Plymouth Guardians did supply some figures for publication which indicated broad areas of expenditure and listed the Union officers to whom stipends were paid. In 1848 the Guardians agreed a total expenditure of £14,450. Despite the intentions of the Poor Law Amendment Act and the best efforts of the Poor Law Board thereafter to implement them, the largest slice was the £7,600 paid in outdoor relief to the permanent poor residing in the Union. By contrast, the cost of the workhouse amounted to only £4,700. Salaries and solicitors' bills came to £800. Removals of paupers and costs arising from births and deaths amounted to £650 with sundry other small outgoings accounting for £700. But it was the management of the workhouse which always attracted the most attention, it being by far the largest single and most public item of expenditure and the one which offered the greatest scope for malpractice by incompetent or corrupt officers and fraudulent tendering for supplies. In the 1840s the Guardians employed fourteen staff. As clerk, Burnard received £130 per annum and his wife £45 as workhouse matron. The Treasurer was paid £97, the storekeeper £60 and there were two relieving officers paid £80 and £70 respectively. All were also provided with accommodation, as was a schoolmistress at £30 per annum. The schoolmaster received £62, a porter £26 and a nurse £12 per annum. The Union engaged four medical officers at £50 per annum each, one of whom was attached to the workhouse.

Behind this façade hid a number of abuses. Burnard's wife was too old by 1848 and had been too ill for years to perform the duties of matron but her salary continued regardless. The schoolmaster only saw the boys of the workhouse for two hours each morning and afternoon and there was no evidence of any education imparted. Yet not only was he retained but his salary had recently been doubled. The schoolmistress likewise neglected the girls, leaving them mostly in the charge of one of the paupers. There were about 400 inmates but their management fell far short of the Poor Law Board's expectations.[19] To keep them docile, illegal payments were made to them which were spent on snuff, tobacco and alcohol. Indeed, drunkenness in the workhouse had clearly become such a problem that in 1849 the Guardians ruled that its occupants should no longer be let into the town, where they became rowdy and caused trouble. Unaccustomed to any regulation of their habits, a group of inmates wrote directly to the Home Secretary in 1850 to complain of their harsh treatment. Gulson, predictably, was astonished by what he had stumbled across.

Redruth in Cornwall provided Gulson with his ideal workhouse. By comparison, the Plymouth Guardians had no hope of satisfying the inspector's requirements. Redruth gave its residents a cheap and meagre diet, yet they were invariably healthy and in good spirits. Being on a hill, the building was well ventilated and properly drained and was clean in every particular. It was economically yet efficiently managed. The accommodation was good and all those who were not bed-ridden were employed about the establishment; even old women were sent out to weed in the bracing air. At Plymouth there was overcrowding with the distressing spectacle of lunatics being housed among and disturbing other people. The dormitories had to double as day rooms and everywhere disorder and dirt prevailed. Ventilation was very bad and the smell was frequently offensive. Aside from these physical deficiencies the day-to-day management of the workhouse was perceived to be poor.

However harsh Gulson's censure of the Plymouth Guardians, the situation in East Stonehouse was in many respects worse. The Guardians of East Stonehouse had long been Tory and by the late 1840s party feeling in the parish ran very high. Political bitterness affected every issue and at the start of 1849 even Rodd was pessimistic about being able to influence the outcome of the elections due in April. Rodd wrote apologetically to the Poor Law Board assuring it that the Guardians devoted much time to their duties and carried an onerous responsibility, while at the same time he acknowledged the repeated criticism directed against them. Their cardinal attacker was, needless to say, Latimer's *Journal*, which could not contain its delight when Whigs swept away the old Tory Guardians and took control. The normally impassive Gulson was certainly impressed: 'this year *every Guardian was turned out of office by the opposite party*,' he minuted after the results were declared. 'We have therefore a new Board of strong political feeling.'[20] Gulson naturally cared less which party controlled the Board than that its business should be efficiently conducted, and on this account he was far from optimistic. The Whigs had threatened to turn out every officer of the Board appointed by the Tories and he believed the political animosity to be so great that they might actually try to do so.[21] This would lead to administrative collapse and a string of appeals to him from aggrieved persons, both of which were much to be avoided.

Ill-feeling in East Stonehouse went beyond political enmity. Not only was the poor rate high but property was assessed in ways which seemed arbitrary and excessive to the inhabitants. When asked by the Poor Law Board to explain why people objected so much, Rodd claimed that the parish had recently been re-rated after many years during which outdated valuations had been used. That was no doubt part of the problem, but it did not explain how the 1,000 paupers necessitated an average expenditure of £10 per annum. Opinion in East Stonehouse was split between those who blamed the Guardians' incompetence and those who blamed the new Poor Law itself. The former could console themselves with the simple redress of voting Liberal. The latter, however, saw the Whig measure itself as having burdened single-parish Unions such as East Stonehouse with duties which they were too small to pay for. High rates drove business and wealthy inhabitants from the parish, thereby compounding the problem. In 1836 £3,206 had been spent on poor relief in East Stonehouse; in 1848 the figure was £4,352.[22] The difference between the two sums was to be accounted for, it was asserted, not by the simplistic slogan of years of Tory misrule but by the increased costs inherent in implementing the new Poor Law.

Evidence for this argument did seem to be abundant. About £300 extra was spent annually on the salaries of the workhouse officers now required. Even printing and stationery cost nearly £50 extra every year. And the price of provisions for the poor was certainly not to blame for rising expenditure: bread, for example, cost one-third more in 1836 than in 1848. At the root of the problem was the fact that the 1834 Act had effectively removed from parish overseers and relieving officers discretion in deciding who among the poor applying for welfare were deserving; the Act had, in practice, made age and not moral worth the overriding criterion for relief, thereby bringing nearly all the old within its compass. Then there was the expense of educating the twenty to thirty workhouse children of East Stonehouse, perhaps to a higher standard than attained at parental cost in the nearby elementary school, since the Poor Law Board set a curriculum and required both a master and mistress to be employed. With their grammar, geometry and astronomy the workhouse children began to feel themselves above an honest trade and instead of labour in the afternoons could oft be seen walking in the countryside like the children of tradesmen or even gentlemen. 'What will become of the working class of society in future if paupers are to be brought up thus?' disgruntled ratepayers asked despairingly.[23] The 1834 Act required an expensive welfare infrastructure to be put in place which went a good deal further than simply relieving the poor.

Whatever defects the ratepayers of East Stonehouse may have ascribed to the new Poor Law, it was impossible to exonerate the Guardians from blame for the state of affairs in the Union. Not only were the accounts never published, but very little ever seemed to be written down. Nevertheless, the Poor Law Board did ascertain that the master of the workhouse received £55 and the matron £20 per annum in 1848. The schoolmaster received £30 per annum until dismissed for incompetence in 1851. A relieving officer was employed and a medical officer, Henry Perry, was engaged for the workhouse. In November 1848 Perry was also appointed superintendent for the prevention of nuisances in East Stonehouse, which might have indicated a serious interest in public health matters by the Guardians but for the lack of any guidance about what his duties were and how and when to perform them. One feature alone spoke well for the East Stonehouse Guardians: its diet for paupers was considered to be the most generous provided by any workhouse in Devon. But Gulson's attention would not be distracted by that. He identified two glaring failings which could never be disguised: a complete confusion over Rodd's duties as clerk and a serious case of embezzlement which exposed the negligence of the Guardians in supervising the collection of the poor rate over many years.

No one in East Stonehouse quite seemed to know what Rodd was paid for and, being also clerk to the magistrates, Rodd was adept at moving his functions and hence his legal charges between the two positions. After the Liberals took control of the Board of Guardians in April 1849 an investigation was conducted and Gulson was subsequently consulted. From time to time large and unintelligible bills had been submitted to cover Rodd's labour, travel and incidental expenses. But what did he actually do other than turn up at Board meetings, meddle with the electoral register and conduct a great body of unnecessary correspondence? Gulson advised that the Guardians should insist on receipts and itemised bills from Rodd before any further payments were made. Needless to say, Rodd was incensed at the suggestion that his charges should be scrutinised and claimed that his bills were already so modest that there was no scope for reductions. 'Knowing how little work is done for the money, the Guardians and parish officers entertain a different opinion,' his employers observed.[24] From Gulson's perspective it was hard to know whether Rodd had really defrauded the ratepayers or whether the Liberal Guardians were engaged in revenge against the man whose electoral machinations, they believed, had kept the Tories in control for so long.

The embezzlement case was clear cut by comparison, although it probably came as no surprise. Opportunities for the misappropriation of revenues were built into the rating system and defaulting collectors were not uncommon. Poor Law rates might be judged in arrears or excused without adequate explanation and although every Union's accounts were subject to audit, in practice the procedures had limited effect. The Lambeth collector extracted £1,200 from his takings in 1847–48 while in the Edmonton Union another resigned with £2,900 missing from his accounts. Seven among the Bradford Union's twenty-three collectors between 1838 and 1848 were dismissed or resigned when confronted with charges of theft.[25] In East Stonehouse the culprit was Edward Arnold, who had been employed as a collector both of the poor rate and the rate for lighting and watching since 1825. It was common knowledge that large sums of money had consistently gone missing and the new Liberal Guardians accused their Tory predecessors of turning a blind eye. 'Although the integrity of Mr. Arnold was more than questionable, and the fact was well known to the late Guardians, nothing was done by them towards getting him removed,' the Poor Law Board was informed. When the district auditor examined Arnold's records, five rate books were missing. The reluctant conclusion was that 'there are yet some hundreds of pounds deficient that never will be recovered'.[26] Gulson attended a meeting of the Guardians on 1 June and discovered that Arnold had already admitted to owing £200 and had resigned as collector. But even when guilt was confirmed political divisions rumbled on. Just as Arnold had been a Tory crony, so the Liberals replaced him with an equally partisan nominee. One local solicitor wrote to Somerset House to protest that the new Guardians 'have allowed nothing but a political bias to govern them and have selected the most obnoxious person in the three towns'. 'The less politics interfere,' he concluded, 'greater is the security for the proper discharge of official duties.'[27] Gulson seconded that sentiment: it was, none the less, entirely a matter for the Guardians to appoint a collector of the poor rate.

By comparison with Plymouth and East Stonehouse the management of poor relief in Devonport seemed efficient. As the Board of Guardians for the single-parish Union of Stoke Damerel, the Improvement Commissioners there employed fifteen officers at a total salary cost in 1847 of £622. The clerk acted for both bodies for a stipend of £60 per annum; then there was a workhouse governor at £150 and his wife as matron, two relieving officers, two schoolteachers, two beadles, a treasurer and a gatekeeper. The Stoke Damerel Guardians took their medical responsibilities seriously, employing two attendants for the twenty or so lunatics in the Devonport workhouse and two parish surgeons at £60 per annum. Their generosity evaporated, however, when in March 1849 they decided to appoint a third medical officer but in order to keep down costs reduced the annual stipend of all three surgeons to £45. They then found themselves with only one applicant, since resident practitioners conspired not to tender at the lower level of remuneration. Eventually three parish surgeons were appointed, one of whom was obliged to attend the workhouse every day in order to conduct inspections.

Like most Unions, Stoke Damerel found it impossible to implement the principle of the new Poor Law whereby outdoor relief should cease. Four hundred souls was the most its workhouse could hold; in any case, as elsewhere, the cost of outdoor relief was much lower. The Union had seen its expenditure on poor relief fall initially after 1834: from £9,129 in that year to £7,770 in 1837. But levels rose thereafter and the figure was again over £9,000 per annum in 1840 and 1841 dipping back only slightly to £8,404 in 1843. In 1848 Stoke Damerel was returned as spending £9,809 on poor relief.[28] In February 1847 the Union's accounts revealed 1,329 persons receiving outdoor relief at a total cost of only £80 – small indeed compared to the costs of running a workhouse. The workhouse was, in fact, overrun with the aged and infirm; among its 381 occupants in 1848 were only twelve able-bodied adults.

The Improvement Commissioners acknowledged that the old building was too small and ill-suited to its present purpose but so much land in Devonport was government-owned and held by the Board of Ordnance that in the 1840s it was impossible to devise any alternative. Gulson's predecessor visited the institution in 1843 and felt that the Commissioners did well in the circumstances to operate a clean and orderly establishment. Gulson inspected the structure in 1847 and found it a miserable place. He could do nothing about it, though, and when reporting to the Poor Law Board he reverted to his favourite theme of how age-old provisions enshrined in Local Acts frustrated modernisation.

For all his disparaging remarks about Local Acts, Gulson was not entirely devoid of sensitivity to local feelings. Indeed, he could not ignore the fact that in all three towns a spirit of defiance was openly expressed. At a meeting of the Plymouth Improvement Commissioners, called to consider whether the provisions of the 1848 Public Health Act should be adopted, one leading figure opposed the suggestion on the grounds that it would breach 'the great principle of local government and popular control, which was the glory of our constitution'.[29] Another Commissioner, who was also a Plymouth Guardian, bluntly informed the Poor Law Board that most of his colleagues on the Board of Guardians 'are most strongly opposed to the Poor Law Amendment Act, and consequently are quite ignorant of its provisions'. He concluded, 'I beg respectfully to say that the general law vested in your Board is obnoxious to the Guardians of this town.'[30] The Plymouth Guardians simply ignored the district auditor when he pointed out the illegality of loans which they had contracted; they knew very well that Hughes had almost no power to enforce his disallowance of their corporate actions.

As usual the workhouse generated the most contention between Guardians and the Poor Law inspector, especially since the Poor Law Board was urging both Plymouth and Stoke Damerel to incur the expense of erecting larger buildings. Gulson cautioned that 'the jealousy of their independence on the part of the Guardians is so great as to render it inexpedient to interfere except by advice'.[31] Furthermore, it was not easy even for a rigorous inspector to discover just how many persons resided in a workhouse. Returns to Somerset House made by the Guardians of both Plymouth and Stoke Damerel suggested numbers in excess of maximum capacity, but since the Guardians themselves were the judges of capacity it was hard to fix any limit. So overcrowded had the Devonport workhouse become by 1848 that on a second visit Gulson noted with foreboding that if cholera appeared half the inmates would suffer. But prior to 1849 outside pressures had virtually no effect on the stubborn defence of parochial autonomy. A major epidemic revealing the inadequacies of public health provision in the three towns would indeed prove necessary before attitudes began to change.

In Devon, as in so much of Britain, debate and discord over the operation of the new Poor Law took place throughout the 1840s against a background of economic depression. Nowhere was this more clearly indicated than in the rising levels of unemployment and pauperism experienced by almost all the Unions in the West of England. The records of the Plymouth Guardians showed expenditure on poor relief increasing from £9,388 in 1840–41 to £10,851 in 1845–46. In 1846–47 the figure jumped to £13,384, distorted by the end of the five – year settlement qualification for paupers in the town, but thereafter leapt again to £16,529 in 1847–48 and remained above £15,000 in 1848–49.

East Stonehouse experienced the same sharp rise: the Union provided for 407 paupers, including children, in 1845–46 whereas by 1847–48 over 730 were registered as receiving relief and still above 700 in 1848–49.[32] Gulson went to considerable lengths to analyse the causes of distress. It was not uniform, he concluded; indeed his year as inspector in central England in 1846 had revealed great disparities regarding wages and employment. Oxfordshire, then and since, had enjoyed good harvests and full agricultural employment. The poor had remained both healthy and few in number and the poor rate levied was the lowest that he had encountered. Coming to the West Country in 1847, however, the difference had been very marked. The quality of grain in recent harvests had been poor and agricultural prices were among the lowest in the country. No further reduction of wages was possible. Farmers had already laid off their labourers to a greater extent than before.

Throughout the late 1840s Gulson observed the deteriorating economic conditions in both mining and farming areas. Metal prices had fallen and the copper mines of Cornwall had been particularly badly affected. Many mine labourers were consequently displaced, being forced to move with their families in search of other types of work nearby or else to migrate alone to the collieries of south Wales. Local subscriptions had helped some families to move; in some Unions migration was assisted from the poor rate as a smaller outlay than providing either outdoor or workhouse relief. Contrary to the spirit of the 1834 Poor Law, Guardians also diverted money raised for highway improvement towards meeting the unprecedented burden of welfare. This disguised the true extent of outdoor relief and in practice, Gulson recognised, provided Unions with a mechanism for short-term support for able-bodied men without forcing the whole family into the workhouse. The same practices could be found across the Unions in his district where agricultural distress was apparent. Poverty on the land was compounded, Gulson noted, by the widespread system of truck, whereby a farmer could compel his labourers, even with reduced wages, to purchase his grain at a price above the market rate. No inspector could hope to influence relationships between farmers and labourers even when they were contributory to the social problem which the Poor Law itself had been designed to regulate. Nevertheless Gulson appealed to the President of the Poor Law Board to bring the trucking system to the attention of his government colleagues. It was a wholly unfair practice whereby farmers effectively used their labourers to minimise their own suffering in hard times.

Truck was not the only blight which fell specifically upon the rural poor during a time of general depression. Even after 1846 Gulson still identified the five-year rule on settlement as a punitive restriction on working men. He favoured an abolition of the law of settlement as, he believed, did the Guardians of most of the Unions in his district. Poor men were understandably reluctant to remove their families from an area where they had entitlement to relief even when opportunities for employment might be better elsewhere. Admittedly the towns complained that the drift of the labouring population and poor from the countryside placed an ever-growing burden of welfare upon urban ratepayers, but with settlement restrictions removed 'the poor man will be set free to make the best market for his labour'.[33] Gulson was convinced that this would at least remove one of the chronic causes of rural under-employment, which he regarded as being at the root of the economic depression besetting the West Country in the 1840s. In any case, agricultural distress had serious consequences for trade in the towns. In Exeter, for example, many of the large shops in the most prosperous parts were vacant despite being offered at low rents. The ratepayers of Plymouth might well resent proposals whereby the costs of pauper relief be transferred from rural to urban parishes, but it was futile to imagine that they could isolate themselves from the widespread economic malaise which afflicted the entire region.

CHAPTER 3

Naval Towns and Naval Medicine

A NUMBER OF ports and towns across southern Britain had a prominent naval presence. Greenwich, with its hospital for naval pensioners since 1694 and its schools for the sons and orphans of officers and seamen established in the eighteenth and early nineteenth centuries, had a long association and Deptford, with its historic dockyard, still served as the major victualling and storage depot for the service. Sheerness and Pembroke both had dockyards while Falmouth remained a naval port in the mid-nineteenth century. Woolwich, in addition to its army connections, had a large Royal Marines barracks and infirmary. But three places above all were always most identified with the Royal Navy: Chatham, Portsmouth and Plymouth. The Navy was vital to their local economies; many among their populations were the families of seamen. Inevitably the health and welfare of these towns were matters of concern to the Admiralty. They affected the ease with which crews could be recruited and the physical quality of the men on whom the efficiency of the Navy as a fighting force ultimately depended.

In addition to the ordinary sailors and marines who inhabited the poorer districts of Plymouth, Devonport and East Stonehouse, many officers resided there and participated in the civic life of these important south Devon naval towns. The Admiralty invariably urged senior officers appointed to port, dockyard, victualling yard and hospital commands to keep aloof from politics, but the injunction was not always observed. The Stoke Damerel Act of 1814 which authorised its Improvement Commission actually required that the Port Admiral at Plymouth and the commander of the Devonport dockyard be included *ex officio*. Past mayors of Plymouth had been naval captains: Richard Arthur in 1818 and 1826, Nicholas Lockyer in 1823 and 1830, William

Wise in 1829 and Aaron Tozer in 1831. Naval officers were also to be found among the Poor Law Guardians, where it was sometimes difficult to keep a distance from factional discord. Too often, as the Admiralty feared, the Tory instincts of many of its senior officers and the identification of their predecessors with the closed politics of the old Corporation led to unfavourable comment in the press and risked ill-feeling with the new democratic structures by which Plymouth was governed after 1835. Latimer certainly seized his opportunity to lampoon the naval interest in East Stonehouse after the elections of 1849, reminding readers how for two years previously an old admiral had been chairman of the Board of Guardians supported by Tory members. Now the admiral was ousted, the election being 'a complete triumph of the parishioners over martial law and Tory rule'.[1] This was precisely what the Admiralty wished to avoid. By contrast, when the Lords of the Admiralty inspected the naval installations every summer and held a dinner for the officers in command, the mayor of the town was always invited to join them.

Most officers who joined in civic life did so simply as respected members of the communities. The Port Admiral, Sir William Gage, was asked to be President of the Union Savings Bank of Devonport in the late 1840s. Wise was one of the founding committee for the South Devon and East Cornwall Hospital in 1840 and Captain John Coode, who had subscribed to that charity since its inception, joined its thirteen-man management committee in 1844.[2] Coode had previously been Captain-Superintendent of the Royal Naval Hospital between 1838 and 1843. Tozer was a benefactor of the Grey School charity for pauper girls in Plymouth and sat on its committee, occasionally as chairman, between 1843 and 1853.[3] Naval men were regular subscribers to the lists of local charities. They also took an interest in poor relief in the three Unions since the families of seamen were sometimes thrown upon the mercy of the Boards of Guardians due to anomalies in the way in which sailors and marines were paid.

After being three months afloat, men could allot a portion of their pay directly to their wives and families at home, but this was not compulsory and even when done it did not preclude the likelihood that parish relief would be necessary until the first allowance arrived. Gulson cited this as a cause of needless distress among many of the families in East Stonehouse, but was told in response that the procedure was enshrined in parliamentary legislation and that the Admiralty was not at liberty to alter it. Though true, this bland explanation disguised the fact that many women and children were simply abandoned in naval towns, frequently having no alternative to poor relief, and that in the event of sickness the expense of the Union surgeon would also have to be met by the ratepayers. The vagaries of naval life became thereby part of the welfare and health problems of Plymouth, East Stonehouse and Devonport. For the trade and employment which it brought to the three towns the Navy had recourse to the charity of their more prosperous citizens.

Plymouth boasted several charitable foundations; indeed its mayor, speaking at a meeting to set up a Ragged Schools Association in 1850, spoke proudly of its long-standing provision for the education of the poor. He cited thirteen schools in the town, admittedly mostly attached to its churches, where elementary instruction was available. Creditable as its schooling was, Plymouth's most conspicuous charities were its three medical institutions, which had impressive records of treatment. The South Devon and East Cornwall Hospital was the most recent of these. It had twelve beds in 1840, thirty beds eight years later and in 1848 provided care for 191 patients annually, including thirty-one surgical operations. This was a typical subscription hospital, its subscribers receiving admission tickets for distribution as largess. It had a surplus of £150 on its total income of £1,700 in 1848 and in 1849 held investment stock valued at £6,434 and owned a house worth about £800. By its own account the establishment was 'liberally sustained'. After ten successful years the management committee aspired to even greater heights. More income would allow not only a continuation of present services, it announced boldly, but would raise the hospital to being among the 'permanent charities of the land'.[4] In addition, since 1752 the Plymouth Royal Eye Infirmary had offered specialist treatment for people from across the west of England. The trustees calculated in 1848 that since its foundation 18,832 patients had been cared for, of whom 934 had been admitted as in-patients. Growing numbers, however, placed strains on the Infirmary's finances and by 1849 new subscriptions were required in order to cover its small annual deficit. In 1848 the Eye Infirmary treated a record 1,203 patients, 952 of whom were discharged as cured with a further 102 discharged with partial benefit. Up to thirty persons could be lodged and fed there.

Mid-nineteenth-century Devon generally did not lack health care for those who could afford the doctors' fees. In 1841 the county's 533,640 inhabitants had the benefit of 597 practitioners – a ratio of one per 893 of population, which was bettered only in Gloucestershire and Middlesex.[5] Plymouth itself had forty-two doctors with further, though unrecorded, numbers in East Stonehouse and Devonport. For the poor, however, the most readily available source of medical help, as in so many other towns throughout the country, was the Public Dispensary. That in Plymouth dated from 1798; other towns, such as Bristol, Newcastle, Lancaster and Kendal, could boast even older establishments. These charitable outlets for advice and medicines sprang up in late-eighteenth and early-nineteenth-century Britain and served a particular purpose where no general infirmary existed, as in many of the Lancashire textile towns. When the York dispensary opened in 1788 it was the eleventh such establishment in the provinces, treating over 900 patients in its first year.[6] By the 1820s the dispensary in Lancaster was treating up to 1,500 cases per annum while that in Preston saw up to 3,000 per annum, rising to 6,000 at its peak in 1842. Within a year of its opening in 1824 the dispensary in Leeds had seen 1,814 out-patients while visiting a further 400 in their homes.[7] Supported by philanthropic donations, the larger among them also provided midwifery and could even offer training opportunities for apothecaries and clinical experience for medical students.

London's public dispensaries likewise increased in number in the early nineteenth century. There were sixteen in 1800, treating 50,000 cases a year; there were thirty-five London dispensaries by 1830. With the growth of Poor Law medical services after 1834, and in particular following the Medical Orders of the General Board of Health in 1842, the role of these private charities began to decline as Boards of Guardians withdrew their support and the doctors whom they now employed came to regard charitable work as undercutting professional livelihoods.[8] Nevertheless, well-established public dispensaries retained the trust of the poor and that in Plymouth continued to be important. By the 1840s it had an impressive record. In the fifty years to 1848 it had admitted a total of 62,723 patients while attending a further 34,569 in their own homes. In 1799 its physician had seen 555 patients from a subscription income of £265. By 1840 over 2,000 of Plymouth's population were seen and prescribed for from an annual income of just above £300.[9]

By the standards of the large London hospitals the patient lists of Plymouth's medical charities were, of course, small. Guy's estimated that it treated upwards of 50,000 out-patients per annum in the 1830s; St Bartholemew's claimed the even larger annual total of 84,500 in 1859. Even Reading, with only half of Plymouth's population, could point to a People's Dispensary since 1802 and an Eye Infirmary and the Royal Berkshire Hospital by the 1840s.[10] But Plymouth had the advantage that many among its seafaring population received the home visits and medicines provided by naval surgeons for the families of seamen and marines. Furthermore, accident or serious illness could entail admission to one of the world's most modern and well-equipped hospitals: the Royal Naval Hospital in East Stonehouse.

Britain's Army and Navy had long provided medical care for their officers and men, although the standards had often been poor and on many occasions in warfare during the eighteenth and early nineteenth centuries both had been found to be hopelessly inadequate. Neither service provided attractive career prospects for medical graduates and, to the dismay of many young men with professional training, military and naval officers regarded them as little more than servants, denying them appropriate rank and recognition. The Army overhauled its medical service during the Napoleonic Wars, inaugurating a system whereby every battalion with a strength above 500 men had a regimental surgeon and two assistants after 1803. Larger military hospitals, perhaps taking 300 cases, were located in the towns or cities from which the army was supplied or which were securely behind the line of advance.

In 1810 a specific Army Medical Department was established, with a permanent Director-General to replace the previous Medical Board with its part-time members. By 1811 medical officers in the Army held commissioned rank and by 1840 a clear career structure operated with the earlier variety of surgeons, apothecaries, purveyors and mates being reduced to standard ranks of Inspector, Staff surgeon, Regimental surgeon and Regimental assistant.[11] Even before these changes were under way Nelson had sensed that the Army was updating its medical care and that the Navy might soon find it difficult to recruit young surgeons in a more competitive climate. 'We must lose such men from our service if the Army goes on in encouraging medical men, whilst we do nothing,' he warned in 1804. 'I am sure much ought to be done for our naval surgeons, or how can we expect to keep valuable men?'[12]

Like much in the Royal Navy, the reputation of its medical service rested heavily on tradition and its glories, sometimes embellished, from the past. In the eighteenth century three physicians had distinguished themselves as men of science while in naval service and criticisms of the Navy in the early nineteenth century were frequently deflected by reference to their outstanding work. The first was James Lind, who published his *Treatise of the Scurvy* in 1753, thereby demonstrating that lemons and other citrus fruits gave the best protection against this ancient scourge of mariners. He followed this by a comprehensive *Essay on the Most Effectual Means of Preserving the Health of Seamen* in 1757 and *Two Papers on Fever and Infections* in 1763 which addressed the causes of yellow fever and typhus. Lind studied hygiene and the use of drugs in an age when bloodletting was still widely regarded as a panacea for all ailments. His last work in 1768 was a pioneering investigation of preventive medicine and tropical diseases.

Lind's reputation owed much to the credit given to his experimental work by his disciples Gilbert Blane and Thomas Trotter, who both followed up Lind's work and were themselves instrumental in having most of Lind's findings implemented as Admiralty regulations. Blane produced his own *Observations on the Diseases of Seamen* in 1785 and assisted in the production of copious statistics relating to sickness and death within the service. Trotter continued the progressive work of both Lind and Blane while senior physician at a naval hospital and as Physician of the Fleet in the 1790s. Trotter's peerless contribution to medical science was his three-volume *Medicina Nautica*, published between 1796 and 1803, in which his discussion of case histories during an eventful career further explored the dangers from disease for ordinary seamen and did much to highlight deficiencies in diet, ventilation and living conditions afloat. On a large ship of the line as many as 700 men might be on the lower deck for months or even years at a time, and these would often make the difference between a healthy and a sickly crew and between life and death for many sailors.[13]

The skill and dedication of a ship's surgeon clearly mattered, although Nelson's apprehension at the beginning of the nineteenth century had no immediate impact. Theoretically, an Order in Council in 1805 gave surgeons and assistant-surgeons commissioned status but in practice nothing happened. Most assistant-surgeons were obliged to mess with the midshipmen and were still denied what they insisted was an appropriate status even in the 1840s. When the Admiralty was restructured in 1832 and the old Navy Board abolished, the medical service was also revamped whereby its Sick and Hurt Board, which had been amalgamated with the Transport Board since 1806, was converted to a specific department under the control of a physician who reported directly to the Lords of the Admiralty. The post had an uncertain nomenclature in its early years, its occupant being Physician-General of the Navy before 1841 and then Inspector-General of Naval Hospitals and Fleets until recast again as Director-General of the Medical Department of the Navy in 1844. In reality these changes were irrelevant. The same man held all positions between 1832 and his retirement in 1855: Sir William Burnett.

Burnett was a Scotsman who entered the Navy as assistant-surgeon in 1795. He saw action at St Vincent in 1797 and at the Nile in 1798, following which he was confirmed as surgeon in 1800. As no one was ever allowed to forget, he had also been present at Trafalgar. He served as a naval hospital surgeon between 1805 and 1810 before being put in charge of medical provision for the Mediterranean fleet. While in the Mediterranean Burnett studied the causes and effects of fever, eventually publishing his findings. In 1814 he was briefly physician to the Russian fleet and then, with hostilities concluded, retired to half pay and a private practice in Chichester, where he also worked as physician at the public dispensary. He stayed in Sussex until 1822, when he was summoned to London to become one of the two Medical Commissioners who after 1817 sat on the Navy's Victualling Board. By 1832 he was the sole Commissioner and, aged fifty-three, was the obvious candidate to head the new department. Burnett proved to be an efficient organiser with a grasp of detail. Guided by his reforming hand, a comprehensive administrative apparatus and clearer promotion structure slowly developed whereby Inspectors, surgeons and assistant-surgeons formed a hierarchy of competent and committed practitioners.[14] In 1849 the Royal Navy employed 449 medical officers, of whom 278 were assistant-surgeons, 120 full surgeons at sea and the remainder Inspectors and surgeons at a variety of dockyards and shore establishments around the world.[15] The largest of these were the permanent hospitals in the nation's pre-eminent naval ports: the Haslar at Portsmouth and the Royal Naval Hospital, which served the fleet at Plymouth.

Haslar and the Royal Naval Hospital were both mid-eighteenth-century foundations. Haslar opened in 1754. The first patients were taken at East Stonehouse in 1760, although it was two further years before construction was completed. These were huge establishments by the standards of eighteenth- and early-nineteenth-century hospitals. The Royal Naval Hospital was designed to accommodate almost a thousand patients; in the 1790s its Governor even claimed it could house 1,250. The number of beds in all English hospitals at that time did not much exceed 4,000 and as late as 1861 was still little more than 12,000.[16] Haslar, with 1,500 beds, rising to 2,100 by 1779, remained Britain's largest hospital as late as the 1890s. Since these foundations were designed to provide for the emergencies of war and epidemic disease aboard ships returning home, there was no expectation that they would normally be full and few of their wards were ever in use at the same time. Surgical cases were kept apart, isolation wards for infectious diseases were standard practice, while patients with other illnesses were housed according to categories convenient for medical attention. Fevers, tuberculosis, venereal diseases and injuries constituted the majority of admissions. Because numbers of inmates fluctuated, even in unexceptional times, the hospitals returned to the Admiralty figures which showed the daily average of patients victualled throughout every year; 1848 was one unexceptional year for the Royal Naval Hospital: the daily average of patients there was 108.[17]

Hospitals the size of those at Portsmouth and East Stonehouse were inevitably expensive. In addition to their medical establishments each had an array of naval personnel, clerks, nurses, servants and labourers to administer and maintain the sites. The permanent medical staff at Haslar consisted of two Inspectors, one Deputy Inspector and two full surgeons. At East Stonehouse the contingent was smaller with one Inspector and only one full surgeon. But at both hospitals much of the routine care of patients was performed by assistant-surgeons, some assigned to the hospitals for a few years while others, nominally attached to the Port Admirals' flagships, worked at the hospitals prior to vacancies arising afloat. The Royal Naval Hospital always held three or four assistant-surgeons. Predictably, many of the more arduous and unappealing duties, including that of dispensing the medicines, fell upon their shoulders. Often fresh from medical school and newly accepted into the naval service, their months or years ashore at so large and advanced an institution were considered a valuable part of the training to become a ship's surgeon.[18] Those who distinguished themselves in the years ahead might one day return to the hospital as surgeon or Inspector. Short of the office of Director-General, that was the pinnacle of a career in the naval medical service.

The Royal Naval Hospital's educational function was not limited to those assistant-surgeons fortunate enough to receive a posting there. Like Haslar, it had an impressive library of medical works, journals and natural science exhibits gathered from across the globe. The library was not only available for hospital staff but could be used by all surgeons and assistants when ashore on leave or from ships waiting to sail. The hospital also organised a summer course of clinical lectures at which recent and current cases were discussed for the benefit of the medical officers of the fleet at Plymouth. These courses, alas, were not always well attended, but continuation with them was considered to be one of the duties of the hospital's experienced medical staff.[19] Over the years the institution became a repository of expertise in the treatment of mariners' injuries and diseases, taking in the serious cases which could not be cured or operated upon aboard ship or which were referred by the resident surgeons at the Devonport dockyard and the Plymouth Royal Marine Infirmary. Inevitably, such an important institution, maintained by the taxpayer from the Admiralty estimates for the benefit of those who defended the nation, had to be safeguarded. To that end there were voluminous regulations about how the hospital was to be governed.

The Admiralty appointed senior officers as Governors for its hospitals: after 1832 incumbents bore the title of Captain-Superintendent. It was their duty to enforce Admiralty orders and to issue directions for the proper administration of the establishment and the welfare of its inmates. The Governor's remit did not extend to prescribing or supervising medical treatment, which was the responsibility of the medical Inspector and his staff of surgeons. There were, however, few concessions to civilian life. Both naval and medical staff wore uniforms and naval regulations prevailed throughout. Most hospital Governors were jealous of their command and conscious of the peculiar nature of the institutions entrusted to them: that at East Stonehouse observed proudly in 1849 that 'the *Union flag constantly* flies over the walls of this hospital to show that it is a *military* establishment and that all the seamen and marines in it belonging to ships or to the barracks are subject to naval and military discipline'.[20] The history of this hospital was dominated by the reputation of a predecessor, Captain Richard Creyke, who held the post between 1795 and 1826. Creyke had run the hospital like a man of war. He was a hero in the eyes of his successors and of all the lieutenants who assisted the Governors in their daily duties. Needless to say, the medical staff viewed Creyke's legacy with more mixed feelings.

While the strict regimentation of the naval hospitals provided medical staff with a secure and orderly environment in which to conduct their professional work, it also inevitably produced areas of conflict where naval and medical responsibilities were not easily distinguished. The care of patients, for instance, could involve more than simply medical judgement. The Governor and his lieutenants entered the wards in order to be able to assure the Admiralty that valiant officers and seamen were properly provided for in their time of need. Orderly routine, cleanliness and appropriate behaviour, especially among the junior medical staff, were all matters for which the Governor was, in the last resort, accountable. Another area of conflict between naval discipline and medical opinion was that of invaliding from the service. This was ultimately a decision for commanding officers, but taken after recommendations from naval surgeons. Naval men, however, were instinctively suspicious that medical judgements were too easily influenced by the claims of men seeking pensionable discharges or that illness could be used to circumvent the application of discipline.

Predictably, in response to any criticism or impositions from naval officers, ships' surgeons and the medical staff in the hospitals withdrew into the bastions of scientific expertise and professional integrity. They were not to be taken as gullible fools who could not differentiate between genuine and feigned malady or judge whether a man was any longer physically fit to serve his Queen and country on the high seas. Creyke and Trotter had famously clashed over the issue of invaliding during their time together at the Royal Naval Hospital in 1800, and although the return of peace and the demands of a smaller navy had since made the issue less compelling, none the less important principles were always quick to surface on this as on any other matter where the Admiralty allowed a joint responsibility to operate. Hospital admission was a further potential source of dispute: much depended on definitions and opinion in circumstances which the Admiralty could not always foresee.

Given the expense of maintaining the naval hospitals, Governors, medical Inspectors and the Director-General at the Admiralty all agreed that eligibility for admission had to be stringently enforced. Applying the rules to individual cases, however, was not always so straightforward. Some medical Inspectors took a more relaxed attitude than others when needy applicants were presented. Governors might equally favour naval officers either known personally or of good repute from whose speedy restoration to health the service would benefit, even if hospital treatment was not strictly required. Burnett, ever vigilant for any improper charge against his Medical Department, believed he had uncovered one such case in 1844 when Lieutenant Robert Atkinson of HMS *Volage* had been accepted at East Stonehouse. 'Their Lordships are by no means satisfied that his illness was of sufficient importance to have admitted him into the hospital as a patient,' Burnett wrote stiffly to the Captain-Superintendent. 'I consider it a case which ought to have been treated on board.' It was never made clear quite how Atkinson had been taken in or for what specific treatment and Burnett was mollified only when the Inspector, his life-long friend, Sir David Dickson, wrote to suggest that Atkinson's mental state also had to be taken into account.[21]

Favouritism might also involve placing an officer in a room reserved for those of more senior rank. From the hospital's returns in 1844 Burnett caught the fact that a lieutenant was occupying a place appropriate for captains and commanders. On this occasion the hospital escaped censure only because the Captain-Superintendent was able to argue, rather feebly, that in midwinter an economy in heating had thereby been achieved. Distrustful to the last, Burnett persuaded the Board of Admiralty to warn that this case must not form a precedent. 'To obviate anything of the kind in future,' he added, 'their Lordships will take measures for increasing the warmth of the wards.'[22]

Sailors and marines or former seamen whose injuries or illness had been incurred while in the service naturally all qualified for hospital admission.[23] But the Royal Navy employed many other men whose status was less certain. Dockyard workers received the attention of the dockyard surgeons, but did not necessarily qualify for the naval hospitals. In the 1830s, however, East Stonehouse had a reputation for lax admissions and Burnett's suspicions were aroused by the numerous applications for entry. When assessing illness or injury, inevitably much hinged on what the hospital authorities were prepared to believe. In May 1839 Burnett was convinced that he had discovered a marine private admitted for a disease which even the hospital records failed to suggest made him eligible. Burnett took the matter straight to the Board of Admiralty, complaining that the Royal Naval Hospital seemed too credulous in treating the local population, who should more properly seek help from charitable foundations. He had tried to curtail the stream of entries to the Royal Naval Hospital in recent years, he explained, for if all applications were complied with it 'would soon make the hospital an asylum for paupers'.[24] But borderline cases would always arise. Nine years later Burnett warned again that without strict controls on entry 'the hospitals would soon become overgrown Poor Houses' and advised that a recent applicant with no obvious claim 'should therefore be taken care of by Parochial authorities, it being their duty to do so'.[25] In 1849 the Captain-Superintendent and medical Inspector disagreed over whether a watchman employed by the hospital qualified as a servant of the establishment according to Admiralty definition. That dispute, however, mattered little in the end. The Inspector took him anyway in light of his serious condition and by the time the correspondence reached London a course of treatment was well under way.

Just as Governors of naval hospitals were important in setting standards for running their institutions so medical Inspectors could be vital appointments in clinical matters and for maintaining good relations between medical staff and the naval authorities. All medical appointments, from Inspector to assistant-surgeon, were the prerogative of the Director-General by way of formal recommendation to the Board of Admiralty. The Royal Naval Hospital enjoyed long years of relative calm during Dickson's time between 1824 and 1847. Undoubtedly Dickson took too generous a view on admissions, but he was a well-respected figure and a tactful handler of naval personnel. His successor, Robert Armstrong, was a disaster whose conduct with respect to victualling procurement brought both the hospital and the Medical Department into disrepute and whom Burnett eventually persuaded the Admiralty to dismiss in January 1849, following an official enquiry.

Armstrong did not go quietly and the scandal, as the local press gleefully observed, became the talk of Plymouth, Devonport and East Stonehouse. In need of a man who could restore equilibrium at the hospital and repair the damage done, Burnett turned to another of his old friends: William Rae.

Like Dickson and Burnett, Rae was among the many Scotsmen who entered the Navy's service having received their medical qualifications from Scottish universities. In the bizarre circumstances of his promotion to East Stonehouse Rae was a safe pair of hands whose judgement could be trusted and whose diligence and clinical experience were beyond question. Rae served during the French wars, having entered in 1805 and been confirmed as full surgeon in 1808. He had earned much praise for his success in limiting the ravages of yellow fever in the fleet at Gibraltar in 1813.[26] He served for years with distinction as surgeon at the Melville naval hospital in Chatham, where he was given medical charge in 1840 and promoted to Deputy Inspector. Burnett noted in 1843 that Chatham was invariably more sickly than other naval towns; nevertheless, Rae had undoubtedly raised the standards of care available there and Burnett felt able to assure the Admiralty that 'amongst our naval hospitals, Melville hospital is equal to any now existing and is a credit to the service'.[27] Seniority and an impressive professional record were unquestionably assets which Rae brought to East Stonehouse; within weeks of taking up his new duties, however, events were to prove that much more than medical expertise would be required.

CHAPTER 4

The Advent of Cholera

CHOLERA WAS NOT new to Plymouth in 1849. Neither the south Devon towns nor the other naval communities at Chatham, Sheerness, Woolwich or Portsmouth had been spared Britain's first epidemic in 1831–32. At Chatham, where the incidence of disease was particularly severe among convicts, one of the Navy's hulks had to be converted into a cholera hospital for prisoners while another vessel was supplied soon after in preparation for the anticipated influx of patients from the dockyard and from sailors both living in the neighbourhood and aboard ships at anchor. Within a week almost a hundred cholera cases had been taken aboard, of whom twenty had died. In June 1832 two assistants were despatched from Haslar to help on the hospital ship in the Medway and in July a further assistant was assigned to one of the convict hulks after the regular surgeon had collapsed from fatigue. Worse still, cholera was diagnosed in the Royal Marines barracks in Chatham, having already claimed several lives in those quarters of the town where most of the married men resided. An extra assistant-surgeon arrived at the Royal Marine Infirmary in July to join in the laborious task of visiting the houses of sick men and their families.

Although the epidemic lasted only about six weeks, Chatham in 1832 revealed starkly the problems in tackling the disease. First, treatment was labour-intensive. Extra assistants assigned to hospital ships and infirmaries undoubtedly helped, but qualified medical men were never likely to be available in sufficient numbers to provide the constant nursing care upon which the recovery of the seriously afflicted most depended. This meant that after an initial visit from a surgeon or assistant care of sick sailors or marines and their families was delegated to attendants of questionable competence. Some of the families could be taken into the barracks where they were more accessible for medical supervision, but for the remainder the surgeon admitted frankly that there was no hope of adequate provision. He advised the commanding officer of the marine battalion that 'application be made to the Guardians of the poor to send medical aid to the wives and children of marines that may hereafter be taken ill in the town'.[1] It by no means followed that, having located the sick among the naval community, help was on its way.

Yet gaining compliance with what assistance could be afforded was equally problematic. Logic dictated that if medical care could not reach those entitled to it in their homes then the answer was to bring the afflicted to centres where attention could be made available: this was the plan for coping with large numbers of victims among the sailors and dockyard workers of Chatham. But the men were reluctant to come and the result, predictably, was that many avoided treatment until it was too late. One such case was that of a labourer in the Deptford victualling yard whose condition worsened in April 1832 when he refused the medicines prescribed by the parish doctor. The surgeon at the yard strongly advised that the patient be moved to the cholera hospital, but his wife refused to allow it. Complaints of this nature from medics were understandable, although that did not automatically mean that those who entrusted their health to qualified men fared any better than those who did not. One old naval surgeon at Chatham replied dismissively to Burnett's advice about medicines appropriate for cholera cases. Work in Glasgow in 1831 had convinced him that they were all 'worse than nothing' and Burnett need not trouble to send him any further supplies.[2] Most colleagues were neither so bold nor so open in admitting that their science was of little value. The surgeon at the Royal Marine Infirmary at Woolwich, however, was another who acknowledged reality. He had visited the London and Borough cholera hospitals and the convict ships in the Thames as well as tended to the dying in his own wards. 'Medicine in such a case is futile,' he wrote disarmingly, 'and medical men but spectators.'[3]

Useless as Burnett's recommended medicines in 1832 may have been, as head of the naval medical service he was prominent in the campaign to arrest the spread of cholera. To its credit, the government acted swiftly when first threatened with an epidemic in 1831, consulting at once the President of the Royal College of Physicians and then creating a national Board of Health to which both Burnett and his counterpart from the Army were appointed. The Board had eleven members, whose duties were to gather and disseminate information about the nature and treatment of cholera and to monitor its transmission. There was no consensus, however, how best to proceed. Contagionists among the experts favoured restrictions on the movement of population whereby infected areas of the country might be isolated. But this was not practical and when the Board of Health was reconstituted towards the end of the year all mention of quarantine was discreetly dropped. One novel idea did emerge. It was recommended that every parish should form its own temporary Board of Health, the membership of which would comprise magistrates, clergy, medical practitioners and prominent residents. Tackling the disease at this level was always likely to be most effective. Much would hinge, though, on what powers were vested in these Boards.[4]

Local Boards of Health provided welcome opportunities for public health campaigners to press their cause and the powers conferred upon them did represent a modest advance. Boards drew together men of property and standing in their communities and were not simply the officers of other local government structures operating under a different name. In 1831–32 approximately 1,200 such Boards came into being across the land, all with authority vested in them by the Privy Council as exercised via directions from the Central Board of Health in London. On paper they could open and cleanse drains and sewers, cause public health nuisances to be removed from private properties, designate burial grounds and engage medical practitioners who would tend the sick poor in their homes. They could even establish temporary cholera hospitals and were sanctioned to raise rate money for legitimate expenditure.

Beneficial as their influence was in many parishes, these Boards had two great weaknesses which left them largely ineffective as mechanisms for introducing widespread public health reform. First, they had no jurisdiction where Local Acts of Parliament had already entrusted responsibility to Improvement Commissioners. They could also act in practice only if vestries approved their plans, since the legal mechanism for bypassing vestry objection was a time-consuming appeal to the Privy Council for additional powers. Second, performing their duties depended heavily on obtaining the consent of residents. Where owners of private property refused admission to land or buildings the apparatus of nuisance removal ground swiftly to a halt. Furthermore, residents frequently objected to the erection of a cholera hospital nearby, which made the Board reliant upon old barracks, factories, storehouses or other often unsuitable buildings becoming available. To be effective in a time of crisis local Boards of Health needed to be armed with powers of compulsion that could be rapidly enforced. This was neither the case in 1831–32 nor would it be again in 1848–49 when, in legal dispute, the balance of advantage remained in favour of the rights of individual proprietors.[5] The Central Board of Health employed sixteen inspectors whose task it was to tour the regions and supervise the implementation of government directives. So small a number meant that most parochial Boards of Health in 1831–32 operated largely as they saw fit and as the time and energies of their voluntary members permitted.

Limitations on the powers of Boards of Health were not the only obstacles to an effective response to the outbreak of cholera. Notification of the disease was often unforthcoming as the adverse publicity which resulted was invariably damaging to trade and economic interests. In many towns medical men were part of the wall of silence which confronted inspectors from London and meddling reformers: doctors had a responsibility to prevent unnecessary panic and might additionally be pressured by the merchants and commercial men who employed them at the Boards of Health to suppress or delay the reporting of damaging data. Among the labourers who died at the Deptford victualling yard in 1832 was one whose symptoms were obvious to all except, incredibly, the private practitioner who had treated him. The yard surgeon wrote furiously to Burnett that it was as clear a case of cholera as he had ever seen 'although Mr. Wright, the medical gentleman who was in attendance, might not admit it'.[6] Similar denials certainly occurred in Sunderland, Newcastle and Manchester in 1831 and in many places were overcome only when the wealthier inhabitants were seen to be evacuating the town or when the number of cases became so great that a cover-up was futile. The press, from similar considerations, was sometimes also party to the conspiracy. It was not until a month after the first cholera case was diagnosed in Plymouth in 1831 that its newspaper mentioned that the disease had reached the city. In Liverpool, where 1,523 deaths occurred in a population of 230,000, the Board of Health was initially blamed by many traders for having given undue publicity to a handful of cases.[7] In Sunderland and Newcastle the shipowning lobbies effectively stopped their Boards of Health from acknowledging that cholera existed and thereby forestalled any measures for tending the afflicted; it was due only to the tireless efforts of a Sunderland clergyman that a cholera hospital was eventually provided. Wary of interference from distant officials in London, many local bodies, even where there was no conflict with individual interests, showed no enthusiasm for taking steps and releasing information which was potentially detrimental.

Plymouth experienced only a few isolated cholera cases in 1831; the disease returned with a vengeance, however, in June 1832 and quickly spread into Devonport and East Stonehouse and then further afield to Exeter.[8] Statistics were hard to come by since many cases were either not reported or else diagnosed more generally as diarrhoea which, in the view of the surgeon at the Royal Marine Infirmary, Isaac Ryall, led to the extent of the epidemic being seriously understated. As the death toll rose steadily throughout July 1832 Ryall's worst suspicions were confirmed. By 14 July thirty-five deaths from cholera were recorded in Plymouth. On 16 July he reported a total of fifty-two, a total of sixty-five on 18 July and 115 a week later. By then cholera was also in the dockyard at Devonport. Throughout August cholera maintained its hold on Plymouth: 207 deaths had occurred by 1 August, 537 by 18 August and 631 by the end of the month. When the epidemic finally began to abate towards the end of September, Plymouth had lost 679 citizens out of a total of 1,820 diagnosed cases. Its mortality rate was the seventh highest in Britain. Cholera swept through the neighbouring towns in the same way. Devonport recorded 168 fatalities from 342 cases by 22 September and East Stonehouse registered 136 deaths from its 288 sufferers.[9] After disappearing at the end of September, the disease returned suddenly to claim nine more lives in Devonport late in October 1832. As disbelief and panic gripped the three towns the civic authorities and medical men simply looked on bewildered.

Initial bewilderment was partially overcome when Boards of Health were established in all three towns, as the provisions of the Privy Council in 1831 permitted, and steps were taken to employ doctors to attend the sick poor in different districts, to erect temporary cholera hospitals and to publish information and statistics relative to the extent of the disease. The Navy also had to make arrangements for sailors and marines and for those employed in naval installations. As soon as cholera was diagnosed among the dockyard workers in July 1832 the surgeon set up a small hospital there where victims could be confined. The Royal Naval Hospital opened a cholera ward to receive patients from the naval community and those referred from the Royal Marine Infirmary. Despite trying to quarantine infected marines, Ryall could not keep cholera out of the barracks in Plymouth, nor could he save some of the wives and children of marines living out. The dockyard surgeon likewise had limited success in containing the epidemic among the officers and labourers there: he had treated 105 cholera cases by early September, of whom fourteen had died, although to his credit he had lost only five of the sixteen cases placed in the dockyard hospital.

The efforts of the Boards of Health and those of the Royal Navy in the three towns were not unconnected. Although the Admiralty ruled that it would do nothing for the families of seamen currently serving afloat, who should turn instead to the appropriate parochial authority for relief or medical aid, and also that cholera fatalities within the parish of East Stonehouse could not be buried, even during a public health emergency, in the burial ground of the naval hospital, in other areas the degree of co-operation between civil and military authorities was more impressive. When the East Stonehouse Board of Health was formed in 1832, and throughout the epidemic, its chairman was a naval captain, James Maurice, and other officers served as members. An assistant-surgeon at the Marine Infirmary, James Donovan, acted as a medical officer of the Board in one of the worst districts of the town. Ryall was a member of the Plymouth Board of Health in 1832 whose cholera hospital was allowed to borrow fifty iron cradles from the stores of the Royal Naval Hospital at the mayor's request.

In some ways Victorian society was better placed to withstand another epidemic in 1848–49. The experience of 1832 proved at least that cholera was containable. By 1848 a network of local registrars of death served as gatherers of epidemiologically valuable information, scientific opinion was better informed by the wealth of published statistical data and many medical practitioners had worked during the previous outbreak.[10] It was the infrastructure of public health which had barely changed, the 1848 legislation notwithstanding, and it soon became apparent in south Devon, as elsewhere, that the authorities were effectively unprepared for another crisis. Across Britain many of the problems associated with identifying and curbing cholera resurfaced immediately. When, for instance, one doctor at Blyth reported several confirmed cases, no mention of this was forwarded to London. 'From interested motives on the part of the shipowners and others connected with the trade of the port,' a doctor in Newcastle judged, 'there might be a disposition to conceal the occurrence of these cases.'[11] The General Board of Health wrote at once to the Guardians of the Tynemouth Union requesting that immediate action be taken, knowing none the less that this attempt at concealment was unlikely to be unique. Another blatant case of hiding the disease was discovered by the President of the Board of Control, Sir John Hobhouse, while on holiday in the Channel Islands. The disease was everywhere in St Helier, he found to his horror, with thirteen out of the sixteen inhabitants of a nearby house dying within two days of his arrival and all the remaining residents in the street having retreated to a hill-top refuge. In Guernsey, he reported to the Prime Minister, a hospital was itself attacked by the disease and after the sudden death of eight patients there all the surviving inmates were evacuated. Dysentery was also sweeping through the town, yet 'the newspapers conceal these disagreeable truths'.[12] As in 1831–32, detection and proper diagnosis would be crucial to any efforts to stem an epidemic. As in 1831–32 also, no one wanted cholera hospitals or houses of refuge adjacent to their own properties, thereby frustrating even those Boards of Health which were prepared to admit that the disease had arrived.

Reluctance to acknowledge cases in 1848 was entirely consistent with a lack of readiness to meet a fresh epidemic. Cholera had been spreading across Europe again for several years yet, as the President of the College of Physicians in Edinburgh wrote confidentially to Chadwick in October 1848, 'its slow progress on the continent led us here, as it seems to have also led you all in London, to be slow to believe that any great preparation would be necessary'.[13] In Edinburgh, as in so many other cities by the end of 1848, the authorities had a rude awakening. Amid serious flooding in south Yorkshire in the autumn of 1848 cholera was also apprehended in the vicinity of Doncaster, yet, as another of Chadwick's correspondents complained, the conditions for an epidemic were as rife as they had been sixteen years previously. Worse still, his cottagers refused to clean away the filth from around their dwellings even when, as their landlord, he urged them to do so. Whatever the law provided for, he warned Chadwick, 'many say that they would rather give up their cottages than submit to such tyrannical treatment!'[14]

Inspecting Coatbridge and its 10,000 inhabitants for the General Board of Health after cholera had reached the town towards the end of 1848, Sutherland confirmed the view that no lessons had been learned from 1832. The slum areas were as unhealthy as ever and in the absence of any drainage system refuse of all sorts was simply thrown into ditches or into the canal which ran through the town. Between 9 and 24 December 130 deaths had occurred from among 223 cholera cases; even so, the authorities there had managed to do little more than organise the whitewashing of a few houses and distribute some medicine from four public dispensaries. Suitable school buildings were available for use, yet no thought had ever been given to which might make a cholera hospital or a house of refuge, with the result that neither had been created.[15] Similar conditions were reported from Castleford, where one medical officer begged the General Board of Health to send an inspector both to verify his account of the state of the village and because he believed that an inspector would enforce the sanitary laws. The request was naïve in all respects. Responding to a similar plea from Stornoway three months later, the Board in London was obliged to acknowledge that 'the medical inspectors were at present fully occupied'.[16] In any case, enforcing the sanitary laws was proving to be no simple matter.

Injunctions sent to Poor Law Guardians to implement the provisions of the Public Health and Nuisances Acts of 1848 read well in the minutes of the General Board of Health, but after a year of such warnings about the legal responsibilities of local authorities some Guardians seemed to be as cynical as ever when it came to fulfilling public duties. Cholera did not reach Carmarthen until September 1849 yet, despite all the publicity about a nationwide epidemic since the summer of 1848, the Guardians there refused to act. No medical aid for the poor was provided other than the token payment for attendance made to a doctor who could not possibly cope while maintaining his own practice. The sick poor were abandoned to their fate, an army officer living nearby reported; he was astonished at 'the total want of sympathy in the Board of Guardians to the sufferings of the poor'.[17] But such complaints often arose as much from the confusion that surrounded all proposals for dealing with cholera as they did from callousness on the part of individual Guardians. When cholera struck a town or Union, what was best done and how was it to be paid for? Few seemed to have clear answers.

The question of costs was raised with the General Board by a public health official in Birmingham as the city braced itself for the epidemic in October 1848. Would there be Treasury support for the medical measures on behalf of the poor which Guardians and Boards of Health felt were needed? That had been the case in 1832, he recalled, but there was no indication that with the apparatus of the new Poor Law since put into place anything of the kind would be repeated. The answer, predictably, was that costs were to be defrayed by a charge upon local revenues. As to what was best done by way of preparing for or responding to an outbreak of cholera there was much division of opinion beyond the glaringly obvious advice that the most noxious dangers to public health should be removed. Not only did medical opinion vary as to treatment of the disease, but there was even no consensus on the value of erecting cholera hospitals. Sutherland wrote candidly of the 'fallacy of cholera hospitals'; they were useless, he told Chadwick, and the sick were invariably better treated in their homes.[18] Chadwick heard the same from Edinburgh, where one of the health officers assured him that cholera hospitals were quite unnecessary since the few severe cases who needed to be removed from their dwellings could be accommodated in the fever wards of existing hospitals. Statistics merely confirmed this view in Sutherland's judgement. The City Board of Guardians in Edinburgh had opened a cholera hospital in the autumn of 1848, but with a mortality rate of 60 per cent of all admissions few had cause to be grateful. What was needed were houses of refuge for the healthy, as had proved so successful at Leith, and not collection points for the dying.[19]

Contrary experience stressed the importance of removing the sick from among the population without delay. In November 1848 two practitioners from Sunderland explained that healthy pitmen in the area would never consent to be moved to a house of refuge but when ill would be amenable to hospital care. That being so, a suitable house had already been selected as a temporary hospital in preparation for the spread of the disease. Reflecting on their preparations and responses almost a year later, the Guardians of the Sheffield Union likewise took great credit for their prompt construction of a cholera hospital, which they had staffed with several parish surgeons and nurses. Handbills, visitations of the poor, public dispensaries and a house of refuge had also been part of their preventive policy, but it was primarily their efficient little hospital which had ensured that only six cholera cases in the city had died among the 3,131 diagnosed.[20] Given this sharp divergence of medical and administrative views, not surprisingly many authorities had either done nothing or were slow to react.

But there was often a further barrier to early or effective action: the public health legislation in 1848 was not as good as reformers sometimes claimed. This was not an easy truth to face and certainly not an easy thing to say to Chadwick. But Sutherland, like Gulson, knew Chadwick well and was enough of an enthusiast for change that reservations from him were bound to carry credibility. Sutherland even took credit for stiffening Chadwick's own resolve in moments of despair. 'I told Mr. Chadwick one day,' he confided to a friend in Scotland, 'that nobody had a right to interfere in the sanitary cause who had not *courage*.'[21] That quality was now much in demand for, pioneering as a comprehensive Public Health Act may have been and impressive as the new powers enshrined in the Nuisances Act may have seemed, there remained considerable uncertainty as to the use to which these measures could be put. Sutherland was scathing of the way in which the Acts had been drafted: 'I only wish the lawyers had to work the Bill,' he wrote dismissively to Chadwick, 'and were paid only according to the amount of their success.'[22]

The problem, as so often, was that powers conferred on new administrative bodies did not supersede those retained by the old. In Edinburgh, for example, there were three parochial authorities with a further portion of the city incorporated into a fourth from the surrounding countryside; Sutherland lamented that the city would therefore presumably require four separate Boards of Health. Edinburgh was caught in a legal and administrative deadlock. It had only one police for the ultimate enforcement of properly issued public health directives, yet that force might receive four different and contradictory sets of instructions. Neither magistrates, police nor parochial Boards of Health seemed able to do anything and the President of the College of Physicians bluntly told Chadwick that 'the initiative rests with your

Board'.[23] Three hundred miles away, the General Board was of course in no position to authorise how many and where cholera hospitals, houses of refuge and dispensaries should be located, which medical officers should be appointed, or anything else that needed to be done beyond basic cleansing operations. The legislative triumphs in the field of public health of 1848 had apparently made matters worse than they were before.

Whether Edinburgh's difficulties were typical of large British cities was harder to judge. Edinburgh was famous for its lawyers and their agonies over clauses in generic legislation should not perhaps have been unforeseen. In any case, the 1848 Public Health Act did not extend to Scotland and the regulations of the General Board of Health in London therefore were not always consistent with the practices of Scottish law. Sutherland spotted this problem at the outset: 'The law folks here are as jealous as turkey cocks, and about as fussy,' he reported to Chadwick, 'and I have hard work to conciliate them.'[24] Chadwick was well informed about Edinburgh and he certainly believed that the crisis there owed as much to the activities of lawyers as to shortcomings in public health management. Looking back in 1850 he confided bitterly: 'The Lord Advocate, die when he will, will have a heavy responsibility for his obstruction to the application of the Public Health Act to the Scotch towns.'[25]

Nevertheless, other towns in Scotland did manage to escape the lawyers' clutches, probably because local government structures elsewhere were less fragmented than in Edinburgh and where, therefore, the scope for parochial bodies to shelter behind legal argument to defend their own autonomy was smaller. Scotland comprised 880 individual parishes under the general authority since 1845 of a Board of Supervision in Edinburgh and for the most part regional initiatives seemed possible.[26] In Glasgow, Sutherland was positively enthusiastic about the measures taken at the onset of cholera. Houses of refuge were quickly established, the largest of which could hold 600 persons. Similar measures were in hand at Stirling. In Aberdeen, the solution to legal tangles seemed to be simply to ignore them: Guardians from different Boards conferred and decided that they would create a single Board of Health, 'This they have done of themselves,' Sutherland noted with astonishment; they did not care whether any legislation conferred such powers.[27] Leith was the same: the municipal authority assumed responsibility for street cleansing while the parish Guardians set about the tasks of removing nuisances from private property and health provision. 'The bodies act in concert but not together,' Sutherland observed.[28] Even so, administrative inertia in the autumn of 1848 proved not to be a phenomenon confined to Edinburgh as the Reverend W. R. Bowditch made plain from his parish in Wakefield.

By mid-October 1848 Bowditch knew that cholera was already in nearby Barnsley and, seeing that Wakefield was ill-prepared, had taken initiatives himself. His own house was being converted into a depot for medicines that could be distributed to the sick poor and he was campaigning for a general plan of action within the community. But the barriers to progress were familiar. Wakefield had a Town Council in accordance with the 1835 Act, a Board of Guardians consistent with the legislation of 1834 and Improvement Commissioners appointed under an earlier Local Act. The predictable result was utter inactivity. 'Perhaps you will inform me,' he wrote indignantly to the General Board of Health, 'if there is any means of *compelling* the provisions of the Public Health Bill when the bodies which ought to carry out its provisions are negligent.'[29] He too had concluded that the only way to achieve any of the benefits which the 1848 legislation promised was to bypass the structures the legislation itself had ordained. These were dire reflections on the readiness of local authorities throughout Britain to embrace recent reform and of their capacity to cope with the return of a major cholera epidemic. It augured ill for the West Country, which so far had been spared.

CHAPTER 5

The Local Boards of Health

For the first half of 1849 Plymouth continued to hope that cholera would miraculously pass it by. As a precaution nevertheless in May the *Journal* urged that sanitary improvements pending in the city be completed at once, summer being the season when an epidemic was most to be dreaded. The blow fell three weeks later when *American Eagle*, taking over 300 migrants from London and Portsmouth to New York, put into port with several suspicious cases. The Plymouth prison surgeon was sent to investigate; so too was the surgeon from the Royal Naval Hospital, who went aboard at the Port Admiral's request. By 7 June thirteen passengers and one crew member were dead and a further twenty-four cholera cases diagnosed. The Port Admiral sent a hulk to take off the sick, following which *American Eagle* was thoroughly fumigated. The Navy had acted promptly, Latimer conceded, and it now behoved the citizens of Plymouth to do likewise. No cholera dead should be buried within the town, all cesspools and stagnant water should be removed and all drains, whether in the streets or in private houses, should be thoroughly flushed through and sink traps fitted.[1]

American Eagle, however, was not the only worry. Cholera was also in the nearby village of Noss, where five fatalities were reported; one of the victims had come into Plymouth before he collapsed. Joseph Cookworthy, the physician at the Public Dispensary, warned that it was now futile to hope that the town would escape: all depended on the sanitary precautions in place. 'We have been told that adequate provision would be made to enable us to meet the dreaded evil,' he reminded the population. 'But the inhabitants have yet to learn what these provisions are'.[2] Cookworthy had long experience of public health in Plymouth. He had run the Dispensary since 1816, was elected one of the new Town Councillors in 1835 and was indeed mayor between 1839 and 1841.[3] His pessimistic tone drew an immediate response from the city authorities, anxious above all to play down the scare. On 14 June Latimer joined with them by publishing letters from medical officers in different districts which stressed the healthy state of both the population generally and of the workhouse inmates in particular.

Yet there were signs of official apprehension. On 13 June the Board of Guardians met at the workhouse and agreed that a Board of Health should be constituted which would have responsibility for inspecting the town and removing accumulations of dirt and sewage. That Board would comprise the mayor of Plymouth, magistrates, officers from the Board of Guardians, with ten additional members being either Guardians, doctors or druggists. The meeting was not, however, a harmonious occasion and its chairman, a Guardian for nearly thirty years, William Harris, struggled to gain consent on any practical matter. The Guardians did agree to purchase a house and if necessary to equip it as a temporary hospital, but no further expenditure was allowed. It was proposed that the Board of Health might employ an officer for the next three months whose duty it would be to identify health hazards and to take steps to have them removed. It was no use waiting for disease to arrive, one Guardian argued: employing a full-time officer was easily justifiable as a preventive measure. Others disagreed. Such work could be done perfectly well by the Guardians themselves. Harris, who was also a Town Councillor, evaded the issue by reminding the meeting that it had been called to appoint a Board of Health and that he felt no obligation therefore to take other business.

At the end of a turbulent evening one of the members of the new Board of Health, Dr George Soltau, turned to address the journalists seated at the back of the room. It behoved the press to provide public reassurance and in no way to promote panic, Soltau decreed: creating a Board of Health was a purely routine measure and did not imply that cholera had been detected.[4] Like Cookworthy, Soltau had been active for years in the field of public health and had taken a lead in forming the Plymouth Health of Towns Association in 1846. He was also one of Plymouth's leading Liberal Town Councillors, who had twice been mayor in 1838 and 1841.[5] By way of confirmation, the Improvement Commissioners pointed out that so much had changed since 1832 that cholera no longer posed a severe threat. The town now had a far more extensive supply of piped water, not just to the more populous streets but to many individual houses. As to sewerage, a more comprehensive system had been developed after 1832 when the Commissioners abandoned charging householders for connection; many more streets and adjoining alleys were now drained by virtue of an efficient expenditure from the lighting and paving rates. Comparisons with 1832, however, seemed to take no account either of a localised cholera outbreak in 1839[6] or of a damning survey of Plymouth's drainage and sanitation published by the Reverend William Odgers in 1847.[7]

Misplaced or not, confidence in 1849 that the disease could be suppressed was enhanced by events in East Stonehouse during the previous summer. When cases had appeared the Guardians there had quickly set up a cholera hospital under the supervision of Dr J. Burrows, which operated until they believed that the danger had passed. Burrows later became resentful about the fact that his hospital had been closed and began to criticise the Guardians for having done nothing to clean up the parish.[8] But whatever the merits of Burrows's argument, cholera in East Stonehouse in 1848 had been successfully dealt with. Some lessons from the past seemed to have been learned.

In October 1848, with cholera reported in many parts of Britain, the General Board of Health issued guidance to Guardians of the poor. All should remove public health nuisances consistent with the powers contained in recent legislation. Boards of Guardians, or Boards of Health where created, should then conduct house-to-house visits, especially in the most deprived areas of towns. The poor should be advised on basic hygiene and those destitute or too ill to comprehend should be moved to proper asylums. Paupers in their houses might be helped by the provision of medicine if cholera struck; hospitals bringing all sufferers together, though, were not recommended. The General Board reissued its call to Guardians at the beginning of July 1849, but still in Plymouth, Devonport and East Stonehouse cholera did not seem a pressing problem. From the Royal Naval Hospital Rae wrote that the disease was 'prowling about', but not sufficiently to delay his holiday, which he would disrupt only if the number of sailors afflicted became such that his staff could not cope without him.[9]

Not until the third week of July did the incidence of cholera reach epidemic proportions. On 19 July Latimer published an account of how the disease had ravaged several of the poorer districts in the last week, especially within the wretched rooms of Quarry Court, situated on the Plymouth and East Stonehouse parish boundary. The *Journal* observed sternly that the area might profitably be razed to the ground, thereby ridding the town of the dregs of society whose slovenly, overcrowded and filthy way of life had fostered the disease which now threatened all. By 17 July 364 cases had been reported in Plymouth, of whom eighty-one had died. As yet there was no suggestion that any of the local authorities were at fault. The new Board of Health cleared out and burned much of the verminous straw and woodshavings which served as beds on the floors of the dwellings and the town's fire engine was then used to pump fresh water through the buildings before the walls, inside and out, were whitewashed. Plymouth's problems, the *Journal* reflected, had to be seen in a national context. Up to 12 July, 3,458 cases and 1,335 deaths were recorded in Britain; London had 339 dead and Bristol forty.[10] Plymouth's suffering seemed to be no worse than that anywhere else. Indeed, in important respects the town was responding well to the crisis.

One admirable response, once the extent of the outbreak around Quarry Court had become apparent, was the prompt erection of a cholera hospital for the poor of the Plymouth Union at the edge of town on a site known as five fields. The hospital was on the brow of a small hill where good ventilation was assured and it comprised a number of large tents providing male and female wards, with a cooking area to which gas and water pipes had been laid. Fresh straw mattresses along the sides of the wards provided accommodation for up to sixty individuals and with hot gruel available no comfort or convenience had been spared. 'They are as well cared for as the wealthiest person could be,' the ratepayers were assured.[11] Dr Francis Fox and Dr Charles Prance tended the patients, while twenty or thirty healthy children of the sick poor who had been moved there were watched over by volunteers nearby. On 19 July the hospital was recorded as treating fifty cholera victims in various stages of the illness. Five had died since the previous day.

The Plymouth Board of Health also impressed by its swift division of the Union into fourteen medical districts, to each of which a practitioner had been appointed. At its twice-daily meetings the Board received reports from these medical men and adjusted its arrangements as required. The Board of Health ensured that bedding for the poor in

Plymouth was made available; soup, rice and other supplies were provided beyond those which were taken to the cholera hospital. The falling death toll in the city seemed to justify all that had been done. Nine cholera victims died on 18 July, ten died on 19 July, and then ten, eight, four, three, and three victims died respectively on the following five days. On 25 July the Board of Health suspended its evening sitting, finding that its work was amply done by a single morning session. Its proceedings were duly approved by Dr Gavin Milroy, an additional medical inspector called upon by Chadwick at the General Board of Health and at once despatched to research the circumstances of cholera in the West Country.[12]

Throughout July 1849 the staff at the Royal Naval Hospital watched what was taking place around them with growing alarm. With Rae away, the Governor, Commodore John Toup Nicolas, intervened and asked one of the assistant-surgeons, Andrew McClure, to go out into the slum areas close to the hospital in order to gather information about the spread of cholera. McClure was an eager young medical officer waiting for a ship appointment and, offered this unexpected chance to display zeal, went out at once to comb the backstreets. McClure discovered that in the week since the disease had first been diagnosed more than twenty cases had developed in the vicinity. Worse still, he reported on 12 July, there had been a startling doubling of the number during the past twenty-four hours. He had witnessed distressing scenes of deprivation when entering alleys, tenements and houses no more than fifteen yards from the hospital. The sewers were generally useless, being choked with accumulations of waste. 'Heads and entrails of fish, putrid vegetables etc. were lying about in almost every direction; dung heaps which have not been removed for weeks are close by the doors of the houses,' McClure observed. Worst of all, however, were the privies attached to the buildings. 'In many of these I found the floor completely covered with faeces, the smell arising from such places is of the most horrible description and intolerable even in a considerable distance.'[13]

McClure also established contacts with local doctors. The result, Nicolas noted, was an account of unexampled depravity which placed the naval hospital in grave danger. Nicolas wrote at once to the Admiralty for permission to use a few tons of lime from the kiln of the victualling yard to spread over cesspools close to the hospital and over piles of filth that had accumulated in some neighbouring buildings. This was not his job, he complained to the Board of Admiralty; nevertheless 'I cannot yet get the authorities to adopt these necessary measures, though I have written strongly to them to do so.'[14] McClure's graphic account of the suffering of the poor was passed on to the General Board of Health, which decided on 16 July to write to the Guardians of both Plymouth and East Stonehouse calling their attention to the regulations which had been issued.

When Rae returned from holiday on 19 July Nicolas still believed that everything was under control despite the rising death rate in Stonehouse Lane alongside the east wall of the hospital, where at least fifty people had died in the last ten days. Since he had complained to the Admiralty on 13 July the local health authorities had begun to take steps to limit the spread of the disease. Furthermore, when time could be spared from his duties in the hospital McClure had again been out in the streets nearby organising the cleaning, purifying and white-washing of dwellings where cholera had struck. McClure was optimistic that the disease was being confined to pockets of the worst habitations and that the Plymouth Board of Health was by now organised to deal with the crisis. This confidence was enhanced by his work alongside a retail chemist and member of that Board, Joseph Beer, who devoted much of his time to the supervision of its sanitary duties. Beer had also been the driving force behind the erection of the five-fields hospital and, as a Poor Law Guardian and Town Councillor, was a shining example of civic responsibility.[15] Nicolas agreed. He too had been in communication with Beer about the removal of nuisances and believed him to be the one member of the Plymouth Board who took his public functions seriously. In the heat of mid-July, however, further cleaning in the town was essential if the epidemic was to be brought under control. To that end, Nicolas informed the Admiralty, 'I am anxiously looking for the arrival of an officer from the London Board of Health who will have authority to *enforce* the *immediate* removal of all the nuisances in these infected localities.'[16]

Impatient as Nicolas was becoming regarding the danger to the Royal Naval Hospital from inadequate public health provision, there remained a real difference between the efforts of the Plymouth Board of Health and those of the Board which concerned him most in East Stonehouse. In Plymouth, Harris, Beer and another energetic member of the Board, Thomas Morrish, had shown initiative when appointing medical officers, with the cholera hospital and when instituting house visits in the worst areas. On 20 July the Plymouth Board even resolved that it should be constituted for as long as the present Poor Law Guardians continued in office and no longer regard itself merely as a temporary expedient during the cholera outbreak. By contrast, in East Stonehouse almost nothing had happened since the Guardians had declared themselves to constitute a Board of Health on 12 July. Nor was Nicolas the only one who noticed the difference between the work of the two Boards. On 20 July Milroy reported to London that the authorities in East Stonehouse were an obstacle to improved sanitation despite constant spurs to action from Nicolas, local residents and the parish medical officer. Together these urgings had produced a small show of street cleaning in the vicinity of the naval hospital, but that had quickly petered out – a great pity, Milroy concluded, since from its ready access to tidal water East Stonehouse possessed a natural advantage for waste disposal.

Milroy was a forty-four-year-old physician, widely regarded as an expert on epidemics. He had written articles on quarantine and plague control in 1846 and 1847 when he was co-editor of one of the leading medical journals. In 1847 he published a substantial booklet on cholera treatment and containment, drawing from knowledge gained in Britain in 1831–32 and during outbreaks in different parts of Europe in the 1840s.[17] As part of his current investigation Milroy attended Boards of Health meetings in Plymouth and Devonport and by 20 July had also been present at two meetings of that in East Stonehouse in order to encourage compliance with General Board of Health directives. To his dismay, however, East Stonehouse had not been divided into medical districts and only one surgeon was engaged by the Board of Guardians. Milroy argued in vain for a vigorous and systematic approach to street cleaning. He had likewise recommended either a cholera hospital or house of refuge, as the Guardians preferred, but equally without result. 'Meanwhile the epidemic is gaining ground,' he noted gloomily.[18] He had written to the East Stonehouse Board asking for a list of cholera and choleraic diarrhoea cases reported to date, but no reply had been forthcoming. Milroy suspected that the authorities there had no accurate knowledge of the extent of the epidemic nor any idea about how to grapple with it.

It was not only by comparison with Plymouth that the East Stonehouse authorities appeared so incompetent: Devonport also offered a better example of crisis management. Fourteen Town Councillors joined with fourteen Improvement Commissioners to form a Board of Health on 25 June and soon set to work removing refuse from public areas and whitewashing houses in which cholera and diarrhoea cases had been diagnosed.[19] Milroy was pleased to observe that in Devonport 'active measures appear to have been taken within the last fortnight to improve the condition of the streets, alleys and courts'.[20] The Union had not been divided into medical districts and no medical assistants were yet employed for the benefit of the poor. Milroy, however, was soon able to put this right and the Devonport authorities were even singled out for praise in the press, where contrasts between the provisions made by the different Boards of Health had become a feature of reporting the epidemic. The Devonport Board of Health was also trying to organise a cholera hospital and to find a place of refuge to which the healthy inhabitants of heavily infected areas could retreat or the children of affected parents be taken. As far as could be ascertained, twenty cholera deaths had occurred in Devonport by 26 July – fewer than in Plymouth, although ironically more than the fifteen or so estimated for East Stonehouse upon whose Board of Health the *Journal* heaped its criticism. 'What is the Stonehouse Board of Health doing?' it asked angrily. 'Are medical men appointed to attend upon the poor; or what means have been taken to remove, or even abate the disgusting nuisance which abounds in almost every district?' Regulations issued by the General Board of Health had been utterly ignored. A pitiful example of the inadequacy of provision in East Stonehouse was that the only action possible on behalf of one impoverished cholera victim was to take him in a cart to the Plymouth hospital at five fields. When admission there was refused to the sick of another Union the victim was unsuccessfully offered to the East Stonehouse workhouse and finally brought back to his hovel to lie on the same pile of woodshavings where he had been first discovered. Was this case representative of the medical care available? 'It is very difficult to get any correct facts respecting the state of Stonehouse,' the paper commented sarcastically, 'as the Board of Health publish no returns.'[21]

As time passed and with no visible improvement in conditions close to the Royal Naval Hospital, Nicolas became increasingly frantic in his efforts to clean up the town. He was driven by the spectre of great numbers of diseased sailors and marines from the foulest areas swamping the hospital's resources. Almost in disbelief, he wrote privately to Burnett on 22 July that within a hundred yards of the hospital walls the bodies of four cholera victims were lying neglected and there was no indication that the local authorities either knew of their existence or had any intention to remove them. He had written to and spoken with members of both the East Stonehouse and Plymouth Boards of Health yet, save for the exemplary Beer in Plymouth, no one seemed in the least-disposed to act. '*Self interest* and the consideration of their pockets prevent their doing their duty,' he fumed; the Board members seemed preoccupied with 'keeping things as they are for the *sake of gain*.'[22] Since he felt powerless to halt the spread of the disease, Nicolas decided to campaign for all the marines living outside the nearby barracks to be embarked on hulks moored offshore; unpopular as this might prove, it was sure to act as some check on the epidemic. His despondency was only deepened by a second report from McClure who, a week after his first foray into Stonehouse Lane and the backstreets of East Stonehouse, had again ventured out of the hospital at Nicolas's request on another fact-finding mission.

By now McClure was well versed in the procedure whereby district surgeons were supposed to register cholera and choleraic diarrhoea cases with their Boards of Health and he had made the firm acquaintance of several doctors from whom he gathered anecdotal evidence about the extent of the epidemic and with whom he sometimes visited particular dwellings or the areas worst affected. He had also befriended Milroy and in his rare moments off duty from the hospital acted as the latter's helper. His report to Nicolas on 24 July was therefore an authoritative statement. Around the hospital little had yet been done for the health or comfort of the inhabitants. A few houses had been whitewashed but none of the nuisances noticed on 14 July had even been touched: the same dung heaps, overflowing cesspools and disgusting privies remained for all to see while their noxious vapours poisoned the atmosphere. Disparity remained, though, between the actions of the Plymouth and East Stonehouse Boards of Health. That in Plymouth was now exerting itself: it not only took steps to alleviate the sufferings of the diseased but provided for those convalescing once the danger to life had passed. Even more impressively, in Plymouth a number of drainage projects had been commenced which would bring permanent benefit to much of the town.

By contrast, the lethargy in East Stonehouse beggared belief. No one could by now deny that the parish was in the grip of a full-scale epidemic, with over twenty cases and at least six deaths in the past three days. 'I hope that this, together with Dr. Milroy's repeated and forcible representations of the absolute necessity in adopting, without further delay, some precautionary measures, will compel them to cast aside their present apathy,' McClure confided to Nicolas.[23] Board members could not possibly claim to have been taken by surprise. Cholera had been in Plymouth since 9 July, several days before the first cases were reported in East Stonehouse. Even by 24 July no medical staff had been organised in the parish nor had any efforts been made to procure a site for a cholera hospital or a place of refuge. Most glaring of all deficiencies, however, was the failure of the East Stonehouse authorities to tackle the repulsive deposits on the water's edge at what was popularly known as dung wharf. This quay had long been used as a storage for night soil and organic refuse from Devonport and East Stonehouse before it was collected by barges and sold as manure to farmers in the neighbourhood. On the same quay was a slaughterhouse and pigsties, all of which availed themselves of this waste facility. Whenever the dung was disturbed by foraging pigs or barge loaders the air became intolerable. Nicolas did not need the assistant-surgeon's colourful description: dung wharf was close enough to the Royal Naval Hospital for the Captain-Superintendent's personal benefit.

Nicolas described his problem in dealing with the East Stonehouse Board of Health when he wrote to the Admiralty on 25 July. Things were so bad, especially at dung wharf, that in desperation he had called upon the Admiralty's solicitor in Plymouth to begin an action to enforce the removal of public health nuisances under the provisions of the 1848 Act. 'I have to repeat,' he advised, 'that unless some *compulsory* measures be adopted, nothing can be expected from the *Stonehouse* Board of Health.'[24] McClure was sent out again on 27 July in order to collect more data from the local Boards and to assess progress in meeting the emergency. From the placards issued by the Plymouth authorities, 621 cholera cases had so far been diagnosed, of which 136 had died. Eighty deaths had taken place along the area of Stonehouse Lane alone, McClure surmised, with the largest cluster of over thirty in the notorious complex at Quarry Court. He had been active already in spraying disinfecting fluid, supplied by Nicolas, into some of the most dangerous buildings close to the naval hospital. Sanitary measures did have an effect in mitigating both the incidence and severity of the disease in already infected areas, McClure deduced, but they seemed to do little to influence the way in which cholera spread from one part of the city to another.

One of the principal difficulties which McClure faced in assessing his efforts to stifle the epidemic, especially in East Stonehouse, was the paucity of scientific information. 'I find that very few of the medical gentlemen send in daily statements to the Board of Health,' he lamented. Not surprisingly, Nicolas stuck to his view that the epidemic would continue to spread 'unless the Central Board of Health in London will take measures to *enforce* the sanitary laws'. The East Stonehouse Board of Health, he confided to Burnett, 'appear to want energy, and it would seem, *inclination* also to perform their duties'.[25] His only positive observation concerned the character and abilities of young McClure, who by the end of July had clearly become a great favourite and whom he was commending to the Director-General of the naval medical service in the most glowing terms.

Nicolas's resort to litigation through the Admiralty solicitor received a timely boost from the fate of John Gill, a resident next to dung wharf who succumbed to cholera during the night of 29 July. Gill was a stonecutter, aged sixty-three, and a respectable family man who had hitherto enjoyed good health. He was quickly buried the following day. This gave Nicolas his chance. He met at once with one of the magistrates, Dr James Sheppard, and together they wrote to Allan Bone, a Devon county coroner, alleging that Gill's death was the result of negligence on the part of the East Stonehouse authorities, who should have removed the extensive nuisance at dung wharf about which they had received full and timely warning – specifically, of course, from Nicolas himself. Wishing to avert publicity, the chairman of the East Stonehouse Board of Health, Charles Chapple, and his deputy, John May, produced certificates from two medical officers which stressed the danger to public health from exhuming a cholera victim. Without the examination of a body no inquest could be conducted.

In different circumstances Bone might have accepted that argument: on this occasion, however, he was not so disposed. Bone was the brother-in-law of Richard Rodd, whose comfortable life as clerk to the East Stonehouse Guardians had been so disturbed after April 1849. Chapple and May, now chairman and vice-chairman of the Guardians, were the men driving the campaign against Rodd's excessive legal charges and previous electoral malpractices. Bone therefore had no reason to shield the East Stonehouse Guardians on Rodd's account. Justifying his decision not to let the matter of Gill's death rest, Bone latched on to the condescending tone which he detected in correspondence from Chapple and May whereby they had suggested that the 'unpleasant ceremony' of an inquest 'for mere form's sake' might be best avoided. He was not in the habit of doing anything for mere form's sake, Bone later made plain; rather, he was accustomed to a thorough performance of public duty. 'The coroner is not a sanitary officer,' he insisted indignantly. His job was to act as a magistrate in a judicial capacity. To Nicolas's great satisfaction, Bone overcame his natural inclination to side with public authorities, ordered an extraordinary enquiry to be held at the Queen's Arms in East Stonehouse on 31 July and requested that Chapple and May be in attendance. Nicolas, McClure and John Eastlake, the solicitor representing the Admiralty, would, of course, be present too. 'If I find there is culpable negligence in any person I shall assemble a jury, view the body, and hold an inquest,' Bone warned.[26]

Family feeling and political sympathies aside, it would have been awkward for Bone to ignore a request for investigation from a respected magistrate acting together with the Governor of the naval hospital. They were alleging, as Bone seemed pleased to observe, a criminal negligence on the part of known persons which had caused a man's death; if this were established then the question of manslaughter would arise. But as Bone felt obliged to explain, it did matter how the particular Board of Health complained of had come into being. If formed voluntarily and self-constructed by a Board of Guardians, as indeed had occurred in each of the Plymouth, Devonport and East Stonehouse Unions, then that Board was not in law bound to act when informed of a public health nuisance and hence could not be held responsible for its non-removal. It was doubtless highly desirable that any Board of Health took steps to have all nuisances brought to its notice removed as quickly as possible, Bone added by way of an aside; indeed, if it failed to do so then 'public opinion would be against them'. Nevertheless as a strict point of law, Bone emphasised, under the 1848 Nuisances Act, which was the relevant piece of legislation, the onus still rested with aggrieved individuals and Guardians who, twenty-four hours after a properly certified notice of a nuisance to public health had been issued to the owners of a property, could have the nuisance removed and then seek to recover the cost from the owner. It was thus a far looser authority than that vested in a legally constructed local Board of Health created in the exceptional circumstances stipulated by central government direction. For Nicolas and the naval interest this was not a reassuring start, although it suggested one reason why many Boards of Guardians had been quick to form themselves into voluntary Boards of Health. Bone had hinted that he was receptive to open criticism of the East Stonehouse Guardians; equally though, he had predicted that proving negligence would be no easy matter.

McClure gave his evidence, describing the state of dung wharf and the effect it had on the surrounding habitations. This was endorsed by Eastlake, who had also been there and who drew Bone's attention not only to Nicolas's persistent complaints to the Board of Health about the stench in the vicinity of the hospital but also to Nicolas's generous offer to the owner to provide barges for speedy dung removal and to his provision of lime from naval stores to spread over the foot-deep deposit covering about eighty square feet on the quay. All this was undoubtedly impressive. Unfortunately, however, before he died Gill had complained about a second overpowering smell which emanated from a blocked privy. From this privy a drain ran down to the beach which had necessarily been left open while cleansing occurred. This issue was understandably raised by one of the medical officers employed by the East Stonehouse Board of Health but, to Nicolas's dismay, it was corroborated and indeed elaborated upon by the son of the deceased, who recounted that his father became stricken with cholera very soon after complaining of the drain. This diverted attention away from dung wharf, which Chapple insisted had in any case been used for the same purpose for more than ten years without any impediment to health in the neighbourhood.

Nicolas himself gave evidence, although in practice he could do little more than outline the delays in nuisance removal which even the most recent legislation still permitted. Bone entirely concurred in Nicolas's opinions but replied discouragingly that he could only ask about an individual's death and that it was neither his duty nor within his competence to remedy defects in public health provision. He could only hope that Parliament's attention might be drawn to the inadequacy of its deliberations. After six hours of public hearing Bone ended proceedings with the promise that he would look through all the depositions in order to see what, as coroner, he might do. It was a frustrating conclusion to a day on which Nicolas had hoped to see the East Stonehouse Board of Health publicly exposed. Worse still, the forum had provided that Board with the chance to make a defence of its actions during the past fortnight. Unexpectedly, it was Chapple and May who came away from the Queen's Arms most satisfied.

The extraordinary enquiry was naturally a topic of great interest for the press. However, although Latimer had criticised the East Stonehouse Board since the cholera epidemic began and had never printed any explanation of its actions, he now found himself grudgingly devoting space to Chapple and May's opinions by virtue of the factual reporting necessary of a coroner's enquiry. May was able to use the *Journal* to reveal that, whatever the public perception of the Board's work, he had signed up to forty notices for the removal of nuisances since mid-July and most were successfully implemented. Chapple was more forthright still. 'I don't think I have attended to my own business for twelve hours this month,' he announced pointedly when pressed about the Board's activities. East Stonehouse was unfairly judged by the public, he continued. First, it suffered from the fact that Stonehouse Lane, the source of so much disease, was wrongly assumed to be in East Stonehouse. It was, in fact, in Plymouth and not therefore his Board's responsibility. Cholera had been brought into East Stonehouse from Plymouth – as everyone knew.

Second, regarding dung wharf, not only had it long existed but it had become a convenient deposit for the soil of Plymouth, Devonport and other places nearby. Yet blame for the inevitable consequence of its location fell upon the authorities in East Stonehouse alone. As for Nicolas's complaints about the smell, Chapple stated categorically that despite all the former's correspondence the Board of Health had never received one official notice of a public nuisance properly certified by medical opinion. In any case, Nicolas's wish to have dung wharf cleared of its soil, offal and rotting refuse was quite unrealistic: 'I will resign my office as Guardian and as a member of the Board of Health,' Chapple threatened. 'It is impossible to put the heaps anywhere else. It will cost this parish more than it is worth.' As the enquiry progressed, Bone had perhaps got to the heart of the matter. He asked Chapple whether transferring the waste in covered carts to a more distant field might be possible, at which point Chapple threw up his hands in protest. 'That is impossible!' he exclaimed. 'We must mortgage all the property in the parish to pay for it! To remove it like that would cost us ten guineas a day.' It was then revealed that one of the contractors at dung wharf had sold and would shortly ship away his accumulations of waste while the deposits of another had been sold over his head by the Board of Guardians, which was already in litigation to recover its costs. Matters thus appeared to be in hand in East Stonehouse and the Board of Health's limited legal obligations were all fulfilled. To rub salt into the wound for Nicolas, his associate in forcing the enquiry, Sheppard, was obliged to acknowledge that both the Plymouth five-fields hospital and the East Stonehouse workhouse had acted lawfully when they each turned away the cholera victim who had subsequently died on the floor of his wretched dwelling a week earlier.[27]

Resignation to defeat was not one of Nicolas's qualities; he was determined to continue with the litigation which Eastlake had commenced against one of the dung wharf contractors. The case was scheduled to be heard in the second week of August. Meanwhile McClure continued to supply the naval authorities with such scientific information as he could gather. The incidence of cholera seemed to be levelling off in some parts of Plymouth, he suggested on 29 July, with only about twenty new cases and four deaths on average on each of the past three days. The Board of Health there had identified where the disease was out of control and was concentrating its cleaning and whitewashing activities in those areas. East Stonehouse remained a different story, with access to reliable information as hard to come by as ever: 'I have called almost daily at the Board room for the medical gentlemen's returns, but have always been told that there are none furnished.'[28] McClure's data were forwarded to London, where Burnett submitted them to the Board of Admiralty.

Nicolas drew a further important conclusion from McClure's research out in the towns: the true extent of the epidemic was being obscured. For one thing, the figures did not tally with plain observation: the Board of Health claimed that no more than twenty-five persons had died from cholera in East Stonehouse (excluding, of course, Stonehouse Lane) in July, whereas Nicolas knew of at least three deaths on the single night of 28 July which had occurred on the thoroughfares around the naval hospital. Simple extrapolation, given that most deaths occurred inside dwellings, was a powerful argument that the figures issued had to be misleading. Nicolas alleged that this was almost certainly the case for the Board of Health in Plymouth too. 'Only those are reported as having died of cholera who were attended by the medical officers appointed by the Board of Health,' he warned Burnett. 'Persons dying of this disease who are not of the poorer classes, it is said are not *generally* included in the official report of deaths from cholera. I have heard this from two or three credible sources.' This, of course, put the broadly accepted notion of superior public health provision in the Plymouth Union in a different light; both Boards of Health were playing the same game of discounting all victims attended by practitioners privately, which in the more prosperous parishes of Plymouth would likely be a larger proportion of cholera cases. 'The object evidently is to *conceal* the extent of the malady, as much as possible, both in Plymouth and Stonehouse,' Nicolas realised. The Boards of Health were not neutral bodies. Being voluntary Boards, they comprised for the most part the Guardians who, as local businessmen and property owners, 'are more or less owners of the places complained against as nuisances. Thus their *first* consideration is *economy* and *personal* interests, and to this everything seems to be sacrificed.'

Nevertheless, Nicolas was not to be shaken from his judgement that, even if the Plymouth Board of Health was also fudging its statistical returns, the Board in East Stonehouse was still the most deficient with which he had to deal. Nothing would improve in the neighbourhood of the Royal Naval Hospital until 'an *independent, disinterested* Board of Health be established, composed of persons who have *no local private interests* to *serve* and to gratify and whose only object will be the *public welfare*'.[29] He had badgered the authorities, sent junior medical staff from the hospital to assist in public health work, supplied disinfecting chemicals from naval stores, attended and given evidence at a public enquiry and commenced civil litigation as Parliament allowed. Energetic and understandably much concerned for the future of his hospital and the naval community which lived around it, Nicolas however, for the moment at least, seemed to have exhausted his options in trying to clean up East Stonehouse. But even all this did not indicate Nicolas's full involvement with efforts to contain cholera in south Devon. He had also devoted much time to the outbreak at Noss in June 1849, which reached crisis point in early and mid-July at a time when cholera still seemed controllable in Plymouth and had barely touched East Stonehouse or Devonport at all. Noss meant another diversion of medical resources from the Royal Naval Hospital, which was now beginning to experience considerable difficulties in providing treatment for its own patients.

CHAPTER 6

Experiment at Noss

NOSS WAS A small crab-fishing village situated on the estuary of the River Yealm about eight miles east along the coast from Plymouth. It was in the parish of Yealmpton, one of nineteen rural parishes constituting the Union of Plympton St Mary. Noss had a population of just under 400 accommodated in about sixty-five dwellings. On the other side of the Yealm was the more prosperous settlement of Newton Ferrers. The two clusters nestled picturesquely in their valley, which was ringed with low hills to complete the rural idyll. Entering the village in June 1849, however, all romance vanished. There were few people in the street, the blinds of most houses were drawn down and the faces of those inhabitants visible were sad and serious. In May a woman and her two children had died from the familiar symptoms of cholera. 'This was kept quiet,' the *Journal* concluded.[1] But no further case occurred until the start of June, when a fisherman, his wife and child were all carried off. Thereafter cholera took a devastating toll. By 11 June Yealmpton parish, from its 500 or so inhabitants, had reported 130 cases with twenty-nine deaths.

The Poor Law in the Plympton St Mary Union was administered by a Board of thirty-five Guardians elected from the parishes according to their size. Plymstock returned four Guardians. Yealmpton was one of three parishes which each returned three Guardians. Eight of the parishes each returned only one Guardian. Confusion in the Union's deliberations was virtually guaranteed by the fact that the Union took its name from the parish of Plympton St Mary, which was one of its nineteen components. That aside, the records did preserve a clear account of how the parishes were rated for poor relief and how in turn the ratepayers elected the thirty-five Guardians.[2] Those with property bearing a rateable value between £10 and £50 per annum had one vote, those with a holding rated between £50 and £100 had two votes, and so upwards in increments of £50 until the limit of six votes for owners of property rated in excess of £250. Property in different parishes qualified the owner for votes in different places. The parish of Egg Buckland boasted the largest number of ratepayers, with eighty-two in 1849; Plymstock had seventy-two, Compton Gifford fifty-nine, while the smallest parishes of Revelstoke, Harford and Wembury had seven, seven and five respectively.

The Union had a workhouse at Plympton which could accommodate up to 220 paupers. Gulson visited in 1849 and was distinctly unimpressed by the manner in which the institution was run. Petty fraud seldom came as a surprise to those who took an interest in early-Victorian workhouses; the master at Buntingford in Hertfordshire in the 1840s, for instance, diverted good meat and bread from the mouths of the needy into the swill for his pig-rearing business.[3] At Plympton, quarters intended for the paupers were occupied by the master's own family. Furthermore, food provided by the Guardians for the inmates seemed to finish up on the master's dining table in order to feed his numerous children. This ruse went undetected largely because the workhouse was never full: it housed only 112 persons in 1847, 120 in 1848 and 144 in 1849. As in most Unions, large numbers continued to receive outdoor relief: the records showed 650 in receipt in 1846, 575 in 1847, 544 in 1848 and 569 in 1849. The Union spent £7,153 on poor relief in 1848 from a total rate levy of £8,927.[4] Overlapping the parish boundaries, the Union was divided into seven medical districts to each of which a practitioner was appointed annually for the purpose of attending and supplying medicines to the poor and to extend the benefits of vaccination. Yealmpton was in the largest district, number six, whose medical officer, John Coad, received the yearly sum of £46. The other six districts merited payments between £45 and £23. Stephen Pode, in district one, also tended to the sick of the workhouse five times weekly, for which he earned an additional honorarium of £10 per annum.

Variations in parish size and wealth within the Union inevitably produced anomalies and tensions. With over 3,000 inhabitants, Plymstock might be consoled that it elected four Guardians, although that did not alter the fact that its seventy-two ratepayers contributed about 12 per cent of the poor rate collected in the Union. As it happened, Plymstock also had a high concentration of paupers. But clearly a wealthy parish with many ratepayers and few persons needing relief would feel put upon by indirectly subsidising others in any Union; that problem was inherent in the Union structure which the Poor Law Amendment Act had introduced. Qualification to serve as a Guardian could also be contentious. Property to the value of £25 in any one parish was nominally required, but the case arose of a candidate for election in the Plympton St Mary Union who was rated at £20 in one parish and £10 in another. The Poor Law Board in London eventually adjudicated that the criterion had been met. Most divisive of all, however, was the system of rating itself, which was assessed separately for the property of each parish and which could become quite outdated thereby distorting the relative burden of poor relief.

In 1848 Plympton St Mary was a classic example of this. Within the Union the actual parish of Plympton St Mary, with its three elected Guardians, had a population of about 3,000 persons, spread throughout seven small villages across a thousand acres, of whom fifty-six qualified as ratepayers. But did they pay enough rates and should there be more of them? These questions arose from the fact that the parish had not been surveyed, nor its property valued for rating purposes, for over forty years. The Poor Law Board had given authorisation for revaluation in 1840, but nothing was ever done. The onus for action seemed to rest with two public-spirited citizens, a churchwarden and the overseer of poor relief at the Union workhouse, who in 1849 took it upon themselves to write to London again, claiming that the property of the parish was 'very unequally rated'.[5] During the last forty years there had been much building in Plympton St Mary, lime kilns had been erected, plantations had been made and, most recently, the south Devon railway had been driven five miles through the parish. All these factors had much enhanced property values and many inhabitants understandably complained that the unevenness of rating was unfair and that some now valuable properties were not rated at all. Property owners and ratepayers, of course, did everything to block a new survey. It was within the power of the Poor Law Board to insist on a revaluation, as indeed was done in August 1849, although implementing the order in the face of determined local resistance was a difficult matter. The Union of Plympton St Mary was thus not one of harmonious or established co-operation when cholera arrived in 1849.

Cholera had struck the Union seventeen years earlier. During that first epidemic a Board of Health had been formed, chaired by the Reverend William Coppard, vicar of the parish of Plympton St Mary, which communicated with the Central Board of Health in London. Coppard's parish had suffered most severely in 1832 and following the creation of the new General Board of Health in 1848 he wrote at once for guidance in case the scourge returned. Coppard and some of his leading parishioners sought direction on how best to implement sanitary improvements using the authority newly conferred by Parliament and how best, if need be, to construct a new Board of Health for the Union. This was in October 1848 when bowel complaints were common in Coppard's parish, although no cholera had yet developed. When cholera did break out at Noss at the start of June 1849 there was a sense of surprise. Noss itself had been untouched by the epidemic in 1831–32 and was no different a place seventeen years later. Nevertheless, it was the miracle of 1831–32 which needed explanation. The village was in a filthy state, with dilapidated houses and the street unmade, while pigs and fowl roamed freely as if in a farmyard. But the squalor of rural life was not the real problem. Its location determined that Noss was a public health disaster simply waiting to happen.

The dwellings of Noss were built largely along the high-tide line of the Yealm estuary. A short arm of the estuary ran between the houses, which at low tide formed an isolated lake or mud flat depending on the ebb of the tide. Into this small arm of the estuary the villagers deposited their soil when they could be troubled to remove it from their doors. This practice had existed for at least as long as memory could recall; the original idea had been that the tidal flow which drained the arm would carry the refuse down the estuary and out into the English Channel. By the late 1840s, however, this natural drainage system no longer functioned and the Yealm estuary at Noss had become little more than a ditch or grand cesspool into which the waste of the village was heaped with no chance of escape. At high tide matters could be even worse, since the deposits from the privies and drains thrown into the estuary earlier were often washed up around the houses and then became stranded in the village as the water slowly retreated. The population was effectively living in a sewer of its own making.

As medical officer for district six, Coad confirmed to the Poor Law Guardians on 8 June that cholera had suddenly become rampant in

Noss. Fourteen deaths had already occurred and the disease was out of control. The Guardians recognised the crisis and, acknowledging that Coad had so many other and pressing calls upon his time and that there was no doctor resident at either Noss or Newton Ferrers, engaged William Spencer from Plymouth to render aid. Spencer had once practised in Newton Ferrers, knew the area well and agreed to reside in the village while the epidemic raged at Noss. Explaining the dire circumstances which had made Spencer's appointment necessary, the Guardians then secured the Poor Law Board's approval for the additional costs and sanction to levy an extra charge upon the ratepayers. Meanwhile in Newton Ferrers a committee of prominent parishioners had been formed in order to help the sick poor of Noss with blankets, medicines and other material needs. Most active in their concern for the afflicted were local clergy: the Reverend Frederick Pulling, resident in Revelstoke, and the Reverend John Yonge, rector of Newton Ferrers.

Yonge's brother, James, was one of the two physicians at the South Devon and East Cornwall Hospital who, since 1827, had also assisted Cookworthy at the Plymouth Public Dispensary.[6] The Yonges wrote to Nicolas at the Royal Naval Hospital enquiring whether in light of the emergency at Noss a medical assistant might be spared from normal duties. The request was not well timed. Informing the Admiralty of his dilemma, Nicolas explained that the hospital staff were already amply occupied with 134 patients and that many more would be brought in during the night of 12 June when HMS *Hibernia* arrived from the Mediterranean with what was known to be a sickly crew. By 15 June there were 190 patients in the hospital at East Stonehouse. As Port Admiral, however, Gage recommended that an assistant-surgeon should be sent briefly to Noss. Yonge assured Gage that application would be made to the General Board of Health for permission to engage a further medical officer at Noss, since the combined efforts of Spencer and Coad were already proving insufficient. When Rae reluctantly released one of his juniors from hospital duties, therefore, it was on the understanding that whoever went would soon be back.

Rae did not need to select an assistant-surgeon: Stephen Bowden volunteered and set off for Noss immediately. Bowden had joined the service only four years earlier but he had more practical experience than most young men posted to the naval hospitals. He had received an initial assignment afloat in HMS *Nereus*, during which he found himself put ashore to run the small English naval hospital at Valparaiso due to a lack of alternative medical staff. In the period October 1847 to July 1848 110 cases had been treated there. It was an arduous introduction to naval duties, although Bowden coped well with such an unexpected burden of work and had clearly relished the responsibility. Noss offered him another opportunity to impress his superiors and his initial assessment made plain the scale of the task for which he had volunteered. One quarter of Noss's inhabitants had contracted cholera, with more than fifty currently confined to bed and several close to death. The sick, however, had not been neglected. 'By private charity the sick poor are liberally supplied with comforts and necessaries,' he cheerfully observed.[7] Two days later there had been three further deaths and seven new cases and once again Bowden was quickly learning the difference between performing supervised duties and working in the field with no one to turn to. He soon realised that it was not always easy to distinguish victims of cholera from those with less dangerous bowel complaints. Furthermore, cholera itself did not seem to be a constant: cases diagnosed some days after his arrival appeared to be milder in character than those initially encountered. Bowden's job at Noss was not merely to attend to the sick. He was instructed to report back to Nicolas and for this he needed to produce statistics. Bowden was unquestionably thorough. His description of Noss and of his own efforts there were forwarded by the Admiralty to the General Board of Health, which at once ordered one of its own inspectors to visit the village for three or four days, superintend medical care and try to determine how the outbreak of cholera had occurred.[8]

When an inspector arrived from London Bowden was recalled to the Royal Naval Hospital. On 18 June Yonge wrote to Nicolas praising the assistant-surgeon's work and expressing the appreciation widely felt for the Navy's prompt assistance. 'I am sure,' he remarked, 'that all the poor people, amongst whom he has, cojointly with Mr. Spencer, been endeavouring to mitigate and arrest the severities of disease, will long remember his name with gratitude'.[9] By that date thirty-six cholera deaths had been recorded in Noss and the crisis was far from over. With Bowden gone the burden of routine work fell once more on Spencer's shoulders; he was soon unable to cope. The Guardians again applied for further assistance using the well-chosen argument that Spencer's ceaseless care for the sick and dying left him no time to complete the paperwork relating to the epidemic which the General Board of Health expected to receive. On 20 June the General Board agreed that another medical officer might be engaged – at the Union's expense. The death toll in Noss was now forty-two; 140 cases were under treatment and the village had a problem of what to do with children orphaned by the epidemic.

The Board of Guardians for Plympton St Mary now met weekly, not fortnightly as before, in order to review events at Noss; as a precaution, the diet at the Union workhouse was altered with the introduction of more dry and solid foods. 'Six ounces of meat for each person be substituted twice a week for the pea soup,' the minutes of the meeting on 29 June recorded. The same meeting appointed an assistant for Spencer at Noss with a salary of £1.10/- per diem, 'it sufficiently appearing to the Guardians that extraordinary medical aid is there required'.[10] The Guardians were not resolved to form a voluntary Board of Health since they were performing all the necessary functions of such a Board, and they congratulated themselves for their willingness to incur the expenditure needed to meet the emergency at Noss. Nevertheless, there was just a hint that considerations of economy were reasserting themselves when the Guardians reported to the Poor Law Board on 2 July: on reflection, they judged, there would be no need to increase the amount of meat in the workhouse diet, given that extra bread and cheese would prove an adequate substitute for soup and vegetable stew.

Bowden's recall to East Stonehouse might have ended the Navy's participation in the fight against cholera at Noss but for a direct approach to the Admiralty from the Plympton Guardians. Spencer and Coad could not devise a satisfactory procedure in the village for separating the sick from the healthy and in desperation the Guardians asked for a naval hulk to be brought along the coast and moored off Noss in which the healthy could take refuge. The Board of Admiralty agreed. More importantly, however, the correspondence came to Burnett's notice; he at once recognised at Noss an excellent opportunity to conduct a large-scale public health experiment using his recently patented disinfectant, chloride of zinc. Burnett had been trying for several years to persuade the Admiralty to use his solution as a matter of course aboard ships and in all naval medical establishments. To this end he had directed many naval surgeons to conduct experiments in order to demonstrate its superiority over traditional lime chloride concoctions when removing foul odours and reducing both the incidence and severity of disease. In fact there was almost no benefit Burnett did not claim for his invention, in which he had invested heavily. Used in varying concentrations, chloride of zinc promoted growth in agricultural produce, it cured infections in livestock and, perhaps potentially most valuably, it acted as a reliable wood preserver, especially against the ravages of salt water.[11]

Procuring the patent had been a slow and expensive process since the late 1830s; as early as January 1839 Burnett had complained of delay over 'the termination of the business respecting my patent with my City friends'.[12] Nevertheless, he had influential supporters. The Earl of Minto, when First Lord of the Admiralty in April 1840, was sufficiently entrepreneurial to take out a licence from Burnett for the sale of timber treated on his estate in Roxburgh.[13] Captain Alexander Milne, already well connected in 1841 with members of the Board of Admiralty which he joined six years later, assured Burnett that chloride of zinc might save the nation a fortune and expressed his hope that the Admiralty would give it a fair trial.[14] This indeed happened when the dockyards at Chatham and Portsmouth experimented with treated wood in hull construction and the manufacture of rigging. Burnett meanwhile claimed that his chemical was also fire-retardant, thereby diminishing this perennial fear aboard ship. 'Its good properties only require to be known to ensure its success,' he predicted confidently.[15] Burnett and his financial backers, needless to say, stood to make a considerable fortune.

Although Burnett had great credibility within the Admiralty it had so far been impossible to prove the advantages of his invention. Many naval surgeons reported favourably on Burnett's solution as an antiseptic and an aid to hygiene, but it was difficult to get beyond the realm of anecdotal evidence from men, all of whom, after all, were dependent on Burnett's assessment of their work for career advancement. Burnett predictably described chloride of zinc as 'the most powerful antiseptic known',[16] and it was tested in a number of medical establishments in London and Dublin in 1847 and in the sewers of the metropolis in 1847 and 1848.[17] Further experiments were conducted in Canada in the mid-1840s, where the arrival of large numbers of diseased immigrants had necessitated the erection of temporary hospitals and extensive accommodation sheds where sanitation was perforce primitive and the need for effective disinfectants and deodorising liquids great. But all these trials became bogged down in claim and counter-claim regarding rival commercial products and once again in the impossibility of providing either proof of effectiveness or certification from disinterested parties despite the range of testimonials from civil and military medical officers which Burnett assiduously assembled.

Where independent opinion could be found it merely added to the uncertainty. The Earl of Auckland, when First Lord of the Admiralty between 1846 and 1849, had asked his friend, the Duke of Portland, to conduct tests of Burnett's fluid, especially for its properties of timber preservation.[18] Portland was an eccentric naval enthusiast who participated in speed trials for new vessels at his own expense and who could be relied upon to perform every conceivable experiment beyond those which the Admiralty itself conducted.[19] He devised three different methods with wood sent by Auckland, but surprisingly found chloride of zinc to be the least effective. 'Neither it nor any other invention was good against the dry rot,' Portland concluded.[20] Further tests ensued but the results were always inconclusive; the decay of the wood depended, Portland was convinced by February 1849, on its exposure to the conditions conducive to dry rot and not to any impregnation with chemicals beforehand. The Poor Law Commission had recommended the use and testing of chloride of zinc as a disinfectant to the Board of Trustees of the poor in the workhouse and slums of Islington in 1847,[21] and the General Board of Health in London was kept informed of the trials which had taken place in naval ships and establishments.[22] But none of this was sufficient to establish Burnett's patented solution as a medical breakthrough.

Cholera raging in a contained environment such as Noss had the potential to settle the debate about the efficacy of chloride of zinc and to give Burnett the proof he needed in order to have his product adopted by the Navy and accepted by the medical establishment. On seeing the order for the hulk to be sent to Noss, Burnett wrote at once to Nicolas that 'it occurred to me that it would be a fine opportunity of trying the effects of the chloride in putting a stop to this most intractable disease'. At his own expense, Burnett offered the Board of Admiralty an adequate supply of his solution if they would sanction a properly conducted trial according to his directions in the village. The Board had no objection. Burnett now needed a competent medic, familiar with cholera, who would act reliably under his orders. His thoughts turned at once to Bowden, who not only fulfilled those criteria but now, of course, had experience of Noss itself. Two pamphlets explaining the properties of chloride of zinc and how it should be prepared and applied were sent to the Royal Naval Hospital and Bowden, after studying these, was to take storage jars full of chloride powder out to Noss and begin the experiment at once. 'If it is attended with as salutary an effect as has been the case when employed on board of ship, in hospitals, and for the most foul sewers all over London there can be little doubt of the result,' Burnett prophesied. The chemical would be used in the dwellings both of the sick and of the healthy; it would be conclusively demonstrated that disease could be extinguished in the former and prevented in the latter. If more chloride was needed then it would be provided.

Bowden had already shown himself to be eager. Burnett, however, was taking no chances and, with Rae away, made known, through Nicolas, that he attached much importance to Bowden again volunteering for service outside the naval hospital. 'If the experiment should succeed, of which I have little doubt if properly applied,' he announced, 'it will, I have no doubt, be of great use to Mr. Bowden's future prospects in the Navy.'[23] Nicolas was enthusiastic about the experiment and reassured Burnett that the Royal Naval Hospital used his fluid every day to great advantage. The hospital's store of the chemical amounted to about 800lbs, 500lbs of which was immediately placed in Bowden's charge. On 7 July Burnett ordered another 784lbs for the Admiralty, of which 224lbs was to be put on the train for Plymouth at once. By this time Bowden was already back in Noss, where he had begun a detailed inspection. Nothing seemed to have changed since his earlier visit. A few nurses had been engaged by Spencer and Coad and the salaries to be paid to these assistants were confirmed by the Union Guardians on 6 July.[24] Other than that, Noss remained as much in need of Burnett's help as Burnett himself was of the chance to experiment.

Five deaths from cholera during seven days preceded Bowden's arrival. Within a day he identified forty nuisances to public health and compiled a list of cesspools, open drains and stinking pigsties; this list had grown to 120 by the time he completed his survey on 10 July. Spencer and Coad had tried to solve the problem of isolating the healthy by concentrating on the village children, for whom an old barn atop a hill had been fitted up as temporary accommodation. Next to the barn was a shed containing sleeping places. But these facilities, Bowden observed, were little more than nuisances themselves. The barn had previously been used for keeping cattle and although Spencer had directed that it be copiously whitewashed and lime applied to the dirt floor, the smell within was so bad as to make it almost unusable. To Bowden's further horror, when the hulk *Ringdove* was towed into the Yealm estuary by a steamer on 7 July it was in a similar state and needed thorough scrubbing and painting before it could be used. It was an inauspicious start, but Bowden's zeal was undimmed. He intended to show that cholera was most malignant close to the worst deposits of excrement and decomposing refuse in the village. He would then illustrate the benefits produced by using the chloride of zinc. Already, he wrote to Nicolas on 10 July, he had transformed the old barn with a liberal application; the lime and whitewash had not removed the smell of cattle dung, but Burnett's solution, in the end, had rendered the building habitable. This being so, the children could be segregated and the process of cleansing the entire village could begin.

Burnett conveyed his instructions and expectations directly to Bowden on 10 July. Bowden was delighted to be able to report directly to the Director-General and wrote of his progress in glowing terms. His initial tour had been conducted with one of the Guardians and notices for the removal of nuisances were promptly served on all offending property owners. 'I shall make another inspection,' he assured Burnett on 12 July, 'that defaulters may tomorrow be reported to the Board of Guardians to be formally proceeded against.' Unsure how best to respond to an assistant-surgeon so junior yet who clearly enjoyed so full a confidence from the Navy, the Plympton St Mary Guardians thought it safest to accommodate his wishes. 'I have requested and procured several large heaps of lime, to be placed in different parts of the village, at the public expense,' Bowden boasted, 'and in any case where individuals are clearly unable themselves to remove the objects of complaint, I shall represent that it should be done at the parochial cost.' Enlisting as much of the ratepayers' money as possible in support of the Director-General's project was clearly an irresistible temptation. Carts would be employed in order to go around the village removing dung heaps and other odious material. Then a posse of workmen from the neighbourhood would be enrolled to use the chloride according to Bowden's careful direction. The entire village would be exposed to its wholesome effects, Bowden asserted, while offering an implicit apology that after almost a week back in Noss the process had not yet begun. His excuse for the delay, however, was guaranteed to be acceptable: 'until these *sources* of atmospheric impurity &c. had been removed it would obviously have been unfair to the experiment to have proceeded'.

At the risk of appearing not up to the task of organising Burnett's trial, Bowden had to explain another problem to which he could devise no quick solution: the state of *Ringdove.* The Navy had not put any equipment aboard which might facilitate cleaning the vessel and, needless to say, had provided no seamen to help undertake the task. Gage had taken the view that once in the estuary off Noss *Ringdove* became the responsibility of the Union Guardians. Bowden therefore had to turn to the local authority once again. 'Being obliged to employ persons unaccustomed to the work, and being ill-supplied with necessary gear, she has taken longer than one could have wished,' he told Burnett frankly on 12 July. 'I did not think it prudent to allow persons coming from an impure and infected atmosphere to embark in a ship which was not perfectly sweet and clean.'[25] The whole trial at Noss might be jeopardised if the treatment and movements of its inhabitants were not organised in a scientific way. Once again, however, he had passed on the costs involved. The equipment needed for restoring the hulk 'has been procured by the parochial authorities', he reported, and they had also provided for two men to work aboard *Ringdove* providing cleaning services beyond those which the families accommodated on the vessel might be expected to provide for themselves.

By the evening of 12 July Bowden considered that he had done all that was reasonably possible by way of preparation. Most of the dung heaps and nuisances had been carted out of the village and in only one case of an identified public health nuisance was it necessary to continue legal proceedings. 'There is now not a pig to be seen in the village and all the sties are cleansed, whitewashed, and limed,' he recorded.[26] *Ringdove* was at last whitewashed and ready to receive its first families, though the rush to get aboard was clearly not great. Bowden had coaxed three healthy families to agree to move on to the ship; with their example, he calculated, others would soon follow. He had already used zinc chloride to finish sprucing up the hulk and it had certainly done the job of overcoming the off-putting odours emanating on arrival.

Leaving nothing to chance, Bowden had ordered the interior of *Ringdove* to be thoroughly painted with the fluid before allowing a public inspection. 'I shall take care to compile the various facts and data relative to the disease here,' he wrote to Burnett by way of final reassurance.[27] By 12 July fifty-one persons had died from cholera at Noss. By this date the total for the whole of Bristol was only forty and for Portsmouth a mere three. It was not surprising that this unknown village on the Devon coast had attracted so much attention both from the Admiralty and from the General Board of Health.

With *Ringdove* operational and with all the children whose parents were ill now cared for in the makeshift house of refuge, Bowden instructed the team of six workmen provided by the Board of Guardians on the method of applying the chloride of zinc. In eight hours on 13 July he accomplished the 'thorough aspersion' of about twenty-five dwellings, separate from privies and pigsties. The men used over 100lbs of the chemical, mixed in a proportion of one pint to two and a half gallons of water so as to provide a total volume of 250 gallons of the liquid for the day's work. There was, Bowden assured Burnett, 'a strict attention that there should be no waste'. To facilitate the experiment, Nicolas had sent to Noss one of the Royal Naval Hospital's fire engines to be used as a spray pump. This was a crucial piece of equipment. 'By fixing a kind of spreader over the nozzle of the delivery pipe,' Bowden reported, 'in a few seconds the interior of a small room is thoroughly covered … Complete contact is ensured without pouring an inconvenient quantity of fluid into the houses'. When a larger volume of the solution was needed, as for a drain, the last joint of the pipe from the engine could be easily unscrewed to allow a larger flow. Where the engine could not be brought close enough to a dwelling or where using the hose proved to be impractical, the men were sent in with buckets and brushes to complete the task. 'All, of course, under my own supervision,' Bowden reassured Burnett. The credibility of the project depended on verifiable thoroughness and Bowden's accounts left little scope for doubt that every building in the village received his personal attention. The walls, roofs, interiors, outhouses and 'all foul and suspicious places' were sprayed and his routine for working the fire engine minutely recorded.[28] Two men worked the pump, two others moved and directed the hose while the remaining two carefully mixed the solution and fed the tank on the engine. He had also acquired a horse and cart to carry his water supply and heavy gear around the village. To complete the work would require a further two days and then there would be the problem of the narrow shoreline between the houses and the edge of the estuary. Large heaps of lime had been collected, however, which when all else was done would be spread across this whole stretch of land now thoroughly saturated with the village's waste after so many years. At this point the cholera should have been contained in Noss; the experiment and Burnett's solution could then be judged an obvious success.

But Bowden identified two problems, one of which he judged best to withhold from the Director-General. He was open about the continuing difficulty with *Ringdove* which, though urgently requested by the Union Guardians on behalf of the desperate inhabitants of Noss, was not proving so popular a refuge as he had hoped. Filling *Ringdove* not only would separate the healthy from the sick but would also make Bowden's work easier by evacuating the dwellings. Though odourless and newly whitewashed from keelson to upper deck, the hulk clearly was not an attractive alternative to the fisherfolk of Noss, who seemed prepared to take the chance of avoiding cholera while remaining stubbornly in their own cottages. Moving people, albeit in the interest of public health, was not as easy as he had supposed.

His second problem was confided only to Nicolas at the Royal Naval Hospital; it likewise related to a difficulty in gaining compliance from the population which had the potential to derail his methodical approach when using Burnett's fluid. Bowden had convinced himself on the first day of spraying that the skilful use of the fire engine and considerate employment of his gang had effected an efficient application of the disinfectant 'without inconveniently inundating the dwellings'. This view was not, however, shared by the women of Noss, who were appalled at the deluge inflicted upon even their modest residences. 'Many of the matrons are inclined strongly to resist this 'mess' as they are pleased to call it in their houses,' he wrote guiltily on 14 July. The problem was compounded by the timetable he had devised. Bowden had calculated, probably rightly, that the work in Noss could not be satisfactorily accomplished on three consecutive days and that a break in order to assess progress and methodology should he taken. He had therefore started on Saturday, leaving the sabbath as an appropriate time for rest and reflection. But in the circumstances the women of Noss showed no inclination for sabbatarianism. 'I half dread whether tomorrow may not give them an opportunity of organising a decided rebellion for Monday,' he wrote on the Saturday evening. He had done nothing beyond what was strictly necessary for reaching the interiors of the houses, but no explanation of the public good seemed sufficient to allay the resentment caused. Bowden was sure that he had not been overbearing in his demeanour but, as he confessed to Nicolas, 'this does not avert much discontent expressed in plain language, to say nothing of threats of action for trespass and so on'. 'Plain language', and from so many women, was not something for which naval hospital duties or even life aboard ship had prepared him.[29]

Bowden repaired his strained relationship with the wives of Noss; by the evening of 17 July he had not only applied the chloride of zinc to all the dwellings and outhouses of the village but had also sought out and treated a few outstanding nuisances elsewhere in the parish of Yealmpton. He had used over 600 gallons of the diluted solution, visiting every conceivable repository of filth where disease might breed. In and around the village more than 120 houses alone had been sprayed; when the treatment of other buildings, sties and drains was considered, and the removal of so many dung heaps and other nuisances allowed for, Bowden noted with evident satisfaction that he had changed the atmosphere of the place. Although another child had died from cholera on 16 July, no case had been reported since, and on 18 July he felt able to claim that the health of Noss was already improving and that his labours and the effects of Burnett's solution could properly take the credit. *Ringdove* remained under-used, although the few families which had gone aboard were comfortably accommodated and in excellent health. It was essential to maintain the hulk in good condition, both to keep those families aboard and to render it attractive to others. To that end Bowden gave specific directions to the parochial authorities that every day a weak solution of chloride of zinc should be used in brushing the decks and freshening the air. With the lime now finally spread across the shoreline, there was nothing more he could do except wait to see whether his optimism was justified.

Such creditable caution was not shared by Nicolas who, interpreting Bowden's preliminary assessments from Noss with his usual gusto, wrote at once to London in praise of the judicious implementation of Burnett's plan. So successful had Bowden been in containing the disease that there was no need for him to remain longer in the village. In fairness to Nicolas, he did have independent confirmation of the improved condition of Noss from a visitor to East Stonehouse on 18 July. The implication was that Bowden had been so scientific that he had hesitated to relay the full extent of his achievement until statistical data could be gathered which might prove the efficacy of the chloride beyond all doubt. Of course, it suited Nicolas, who had the needs of his hospital to consider, to represent Bowden's work in the best possible light. By now Bowden had been away almost two weeks at a time when Rae needed all his medical colleagues on account of the epidemic rampant in Plymouth and East Stonehouse.

On 19 July Nicolas wrote again; this time his tone was more urgent and he confronted Burnett with what had become a pressing need to have all the medical staff back on duty in the hospital. 'He will at this moment, with the cholera so near this establishment, be *most useful*,' Nicolas pleaded.[30] But Burnett was unmoved. Bowden would stay at Noss until he had gathered all the information available as to the value of chloride of zinc in taming cholera. Bowden had his instructions from and reported directly to the Director-General and the Royal Naval Hospital would have to do as best it could until Burnett was satisfied that the experiment at Noss was concluded.

In the following week Bowden set about gathering all the support he could for Burnett's fluid. One source was the local Surveyor of the Highways, a former ship's Master in the Royal Navy, who was happy to testify. He had been in Noss before and since the trial and could state categorically that all disagreeable smells had been removed from the village. Removal of foul odour, however, was not the same as medical benefit. The Reverend Pulling also wrote to Bowden in glowing terms about the effect which the chloride had produced in the cattle barn converted into the children's house of refuge, but again this took the issue no further. Pulling knew that Bowden was eager to be able to demonstrate the disinfectant properties of Burnett's chloride, but he could do no more than stress its wondrous effect upon the senses and the great skill with which the assistant-surgeon had applied it. Pulling was also profuse in his thanks for the Navy's efforts to treat the afflicted at Noss and spared nothing in his praise of Bowden. All this Bowden was delighted to be able to forward to the Admiralty, knowing none the less that it was not really what Burnett most desired to hear.

Burnett could never receive proof such as he so desperately wanted that his solution had been instrumental in snuffing out cholera at Noss. It was impossible for Bowden to demonstrate simply from the sequence of events in the village a clear causation; he could show only that cleaning and treating the village predated a decline of the epidemic which might, of course, have happened anyway. Nevertheless, professional opinion could be usefully harnessed to the cause; in Spencer, Bowden had a willing accomplice who was convinced from his own observations that the solution had produced medical advantage. Spencer, like Pulling, praised Bowden for his tireless work in Noss and with *Ringdove* offshore. Application of the chloride of zinc had transformed the state both of the buildings and of the frame of mind of their occupants, he assured Bowden on 22 July. '*Paripassu* the health and physical condition of the inhabitants have improved,' he explained, 'so that in the village of Noss at this present time and for some days past I have had no case of cholera or diarrhoea on the sicklist – a matter not less of surprise than congratulation, considering its condition before you began your labour.'[31] It was unfortunate that Bowden had been unable to elicit any interest in his experiment from the medical officer who had been sent down from the General Board of Health in June to investigate the cholera outbreak. The man had conducted no research, merely serving as one of Coad's auxiliaries and helping out elsewhere routinely within the Plympton St Mary Union.

Bowden's final despatch from Noss was written on 23 July, when he naturally presented Burnett with the most favourable account of all that he had achieved. All those who had lived or worked with the sick in the village had been impressed by the chloride and testified 'not only to the perfect deodorising power of the agent but also to the fact that since its use *all sickness has disappeared from the village'*. He had spent sixteen days at Noss, during which time he had demonstrated what could be done to bring the ravages of cholera to heel. 'I sincerely trust my proceedings in this new and somewhat difficult position may be considered to merit your valued approbation,' he requested.[32] Burnett, he was well aware, had given him a most unusual opportunity to display initiative so early in his career and much would hinge on the Director-General's assessment of his fitness for responsibility and devotion to duty, so important in establishing a claim to promotion. In the event, Bowden had no cause to worry. Reading the latter's careful reports,

Burnett concluded that Bowden had done all that could have been expected. The testimonials and other evidence would all be passed on to the Board of Admiralty, where those who governed the Navy could judge the results of this public health experiment for themselves. They were also quoted in the promotional literature issued for Burnett's patent in 1850, which reprinted Bowden's last report.[33] Bowden was now released to return to East Stonehouse. When he arrived on 24 July 1849 he found the situation at the Royal Naval Hospital far worse than he could ever have anticipated. Not only were its resources stretched to their limits, but the pressures so created had opened a rift between Nicolas and Rae which was poisoning the institution.

CHAPTER 7

The Epidemic and the Royal Naval Hospital

EVEN BEFORE CHOLERA reached south Devon in 1849 the Royal Naval Hospital had its problems: most of those who worked there believed that dominant among them was the Governor himself. An element of tact, beyond the norm perhaps for senior naval officers, was needed for the job, since medical staff were always more receptive to persuasion than to orders and an efficient and harmonious running of the hospital depended on a good professional relationship between the officer commanding and the medical Inspector. Nicolas, who had taken up his post aged fifty-nine in December 1847, had never given much sign that he was a suitable appointment. Making his way in the service, the essential quality of deference had duly been shown, but he was always a prickly man liable to see criticism where probably none was intended – a failing for which he was reproached by the First Lord of the Admiralty in 1838.[1] Pride, though, was tempered by a strong sense of integrity and loyalty to those who served him well: in 1841 he even brushed aside the chance of a knighthood and redirected the Admiralty's attention to the first Lieutenant and first mate aboard his ship *Belleisle*.[2] His character was shaped by nigh twenty years in command of ships on foreign stations, where such notions as delegation or discussion in the exercise of authority held little sway.

Nicolas's brief moment of prominence came in 1843 when, crossing the Pacific, he had landed at Tahiti at a time of diplomatic tension and suspicion that France intended to extend its political influence in the region. However, his support for the Queen of Tahiti against a bullying French admiral had earned him a rebuke from the Foreign Office, after which he felt obliged to assure the government that in any future command he would do nothing beyond a strict fulfilment of orders.[3] Single-minded and with an obsession that Admiralty regulations be meticulously enforced, Nicolas brought great determination to bear on all aspects of his work, although unfortunately he seemed quite unable to differentiate between worthy and unworthy causes.

Observing the way in which Nicolas treated Lieutenant John Tulloh, his second in command, gave a foretaste of what was to come. In case he wished to issue an order for the hospital before departing to attend to his other duties at the victualling yard, Nicolas insisted that Tulloh should present himself at the Captain-Superintendent's office at 10 a.m. every day. He was then to receive the Governor on parade at three o'clock each afternoon when Nicolas returned from the yard. Such a regime was soon to permeate every area of hospital life. In January 1848 Nicolas felt that he had encountered insubordination when a number of patients had passed within sight of him on a public walkway without saluting. His uniform should have made him instantly recognisable, he thundered. In future disrespectful patients would be punished, and he ordered the medical staff to warn them all accordingly. Nicolas next turned his attention to the way in which the hospital labourers swept the paths. A dangerous irregularity seemed to have developed in so far as there was no set time of day for this work to be performed. The paths were kept hard by drainage ruts filled with limestone chippings along either side; these ruts had to be kept clean and any displaced chippings brushed back into them. Two labourers were to be employed daily at 8 a.m. and again at 3 p.m., he ordered. All the walks and flower beds in the hospital grounds were likewise to be tidied and the area at the entrance was to be kept clean at all times. Even in the public road outside cattle dirt was to be removed at once and the roadway washed if necessary.

When Nicolas was not preoccupied with naval discipline he justified his intrusions into the daily routine of the hospital on the grounds of patients' health, apparently unable to distinguish his broad remit from any specific function. In June 1848 he developed an interest in ash tubs and where and when they should be emptied. It should be every morning, he ordered. The ash should be heaped close to the walls of the field beyond the wash-house where, mixed with dung and other refuse, it should be covered over with three inches of earth in order to prevent effluvia. Every Saturday at 10 a.m. this decaying heap was to be transported out of the grounds through a rear gate, which the hospital butler should afterwards ensure was locked. In August the grass caught his eye while observing convalescing patients walking upon it. If too long the grass might retain sufficient moisture to cause damp feet, thereby giving rise to a health relapse among unsuspecting seamen, Nicolas reasoned. The grass should thus be cut by two labourers every Friday morning or as soon after as possible if too wet. Paths across the grass should be kept in good condition by labourers tending them daily at 9 p.m., after all their other work was done.

When Admiralty orders were neglected Nicolas was even more severe. In September 1848 he discovered one order whereby the hospital's fire engines with all their gear should be in a constant state of readiness for use. The hospital had always made adequate provision, but Nicolas now judged that the increased amount of equipment attached to each engine militated against a heightened state of readiness within the existing accommodation. Well-meaning, but oblivious to any sense of making best use of the space available in the old engine room, he ordered the mortuary to be cleared at once and converted into a properly appointed fire station. Bodies would henceforth be kept closer to the burial ground, wherever medical staff could find space, until a new mortuary might be erected. The dead themselves were not exempt from Nicolas's zeal for regulations. Once a corpse was placed in a hospital coffin, he decreed, it must never be removed. Friends or relatives wishing another burial container must provide a coffin large enough to take the hospital coffin too. This rule was likewise justified on health grounds: the less a corpse was handled, the lower the likelihood of transmitting any disease. In the event of examination or dissection of a body the lid of the coffin was to be nailed down at once. Nicolas was drifting into a mindset whereby none but he was capable of either giving or interpreting the most basic instruction.

After a year of this, it was a matter for whispered comment at the Royal Naval Hospital whether staff were governed by a naval martinet or by a worn-out and unstable sea captain who himself needed treatment. By then, Nicolas had also come to see the children of staff families who lived on the site as destructive forces, believing that some were throwing stones through the windows of buildings and otherwise wilfully damaging public property. He confined all the children to one nearby field for recreation where they might remain from dawn to dusk but would on no occasion seek amusement beyond this designated playground. Infringements would be punished in the most severe manner, he warned in September 1848. But all this – although the incessant stream of memoranda and orders was trying for all staff – was comparatively harmless and would remain so while diagnosis and treatment of the patients remained essentially a world apart.

Alas, the wards of the hospital increasingly attracted Nicolas's attention. Medical staff might properly treat the inmates as patients, but for him they were primarily serving sailors or marines under naval authority, and although it might not be his job to heal them it was, he reasoned, for him to provide an institutional regime conducive to recovery. The wards stank, he abruptly announced in April 1848. Worse, they stank despite a former memorandum he had issued on the subject, and this could mean nothing therefore but that a properly given naval order to prevent them stinking had not been obeyed. Specific orders were issued immediately. 'The smell from the water closets was most offensive, and thereby *most unwholesome* to the patients,' Nicolas lectured the medical staff.[4] Henceforth the hospital butler would take responsibility for throwing six or eight buckets of water into every water closet in use at the designated hours of 8:30 a.m., 1:30 p.m. and 5 p.m. The last bucketful of every flush should contain some chloride of lime to act as a deodoriser. As a final mark of pedantry, Nicolas prescribed that the final bucket of the evening should contain an extra quantity of lime. Furthermore, he would not be disobeyed a second time. When the lieutenants on duty entered the wards they would check for smells and summon the butler additionally if required. The assistant-surgeons on duty would consider themselves equally bound by this instruction.

Ward visits by naval officers would also be tightened. Consistent with Admiralty regulations, these had always taken place in the morning, but Nicolas inaugurated a further daily visit between 3 and 5 p.m. 'Those visits in the forenoon and afternoon I deem had better be made at *varied hours*,' he railed, 'so that the nurses and patients might not be prepared for such visits.'[5] At times, Nicolas's orders suggested that the whole hospital was in conspiracy against him and that without his watchful gaze all rules would be laid aside. By 1849 the stresses caused by working with so domineering a chief were causing problems in most professional relationships within the hospital and had, Rae reported, reduced a number of the staff to nervous wrecks.

Rae, who as medical Inspector with his own line of reporting to the Admiralty was the one man in the hospital who could presume to stand up to Nicolas, was of a quite different temperament. Rae was a sensitive and serious man whose instincts were to avoid conflict. His success at the Melville hospital in Chatham had been earned through medical skills and when he came to East Stonehouse early in 1849 he was unaccustomed to personal antagonisms or political intrigue. Nevertheless, Rae was not oblivious to the discontent that seemed to accompany all that Nicolas did; indeed he drew Burnett's attention to the matter when revealing that all the orders of Nicolas's four predecessors over twenty years covered ninety-two pages in the hospital's order book while those of Nicolas in just over eighteen months filled ninety-six. But Rae kept out of Nicolas's way whenever possible; even constant ward inspections were a price worth paying for maintaining a peaceful co-existence.

A peculiar incident in July 1849 tested Rae's resolve. Nicolas took a dislike to the displays of preserved specimens and scientific exhibits in the hospital's museum and ordered all the crania to be moved out of sight. These were educational tools and the medical staff not unnaturally objected. 'When I see him I shall say that we want all objects of pathology placed in as conspicuous a light as possible,' Rae promised Burnett with obvious foreboding. 'Fortunately he and I are still on very good terms.'[6] Returning from holiday over a fortnight later, however, Rae was furious about what Nicolas had done in his absence. The argument about the museum now appeared insignificant when compared with the way in which McClure's time was being used to gather information for Nicolas's complaints to the local Boards of Health, and Bowden had been sent back to Noss for an unspecified period. To make matters worse, as cholera cases had started coming into the Royal Naval Hospital Nicolas had bullied the medical staff to use wards other than those which Rae had prepared before he went away. It was obvious to all that Nicolas's sole motivation had been to accommodate all cholera victims as far away from his own quarters as possible.

Matters came to a head on 20 July. 'He and I have had a regular *flare up* this morning,' Rae wrote to Burnett; he then told McClure that he was henceforth confined to the hospital. 'So you cannot comply with my request which you have resisted in permitting Mr. McClure to go out with Mr. Milroy?' Nicolas sneered when the two men clashed again on the following day. Rae retorted indignantly: 'I could not spare him.' 'The medical men outside were surely better acquainted with the localities of Stonehouse for Mr. Milroy's information than Mr. McClure.' Nicolas flew into a rage and ordered that since all the medical staff were so hard pressed then no leave for any of them would he allowed until such time as McClure could be made available. Yet neither Nicolas nor Rae could afford for their disagreements to boil over into an open rupture and as cholera cases began to enter the naval hospital in greater numbers and as the arguments about public health outside became increasingly acrimonious both men were in fact distracted from this confrontation over their respective duties. This did not stop Nicolas firing a parting shot at Rae by giving McClure a written order to go out of the hospital in order to investigate the extent of the epidemic. 'All this interference retards our duty and particularly the dispensary duty,' Rae recorded; however, 'as I had Bowden I did not mind.'[7] Rae's main problem now was how to treat his patients.

Rae was fortunate in one respect: Alexander Allen, the hospital surgeon and next in seniority, was not only highly competent but proved to be a loyal and conscientious colleague. Allen was aged forty-three and had an outstanding service record, first coming to the Admiralty's attention after the Battle of Navarino in 1827 when, as a fresh assistant, his enthusiasm and success in tending the wounded marked him out for rapid promotion to full surgeon. Much of his subsequent time was spent afloat. He was flag surgeon and acting Deputy Inspector before being confirmed as surgeon and storekeeper at East Stonehouse at the same time as Nicolas arrived in December 1847. During 1848 and amid the crisis which led to Armstrong's dismissal Allen had been a stable influence at the hospital, on occasions even taking charge of the medical staff. Given his credentials Allen would have had grounds for feeling that he was a candidate for the Inspector's post in January 1849, although he never seemed to believe that he had been passed over. Rae's seniority and his rank at Chatham impressed Allen; in any case, the two men had much in common. Allen was yet another highly educated Scotsman who had seen the Royal Navy as offering the best opportunities for his medical education, and he and Rae soon developed a strong mutual personal regard.

Furthermore, neither Rae nor Allen was dogmatic about how best to try to save cholera patients; Allen indeed had experimented freely with their first fatal case on 15 July. Admittedly the victim was in a state of collapse when Allen saw him; nevertheless, chloroform was given in ten-minim doses every half hour during the first day and night. Occasional large doses of calomel were administered, interspersed with moderate quantities of brandy and water. Sinapisms were next attached to the abdomen, feet and calves and then external heat applied to the body via bags of hot sand and frequent friction. Allen had also tried a saline cure, which at the end the patient himself asked be discontinued. Rae too approved of chloroform and measures of brandy. Like Allen he applied external heat and vigorous rubbing of the limbs, but he favoured too the use of enemas preceding a carminative to stay the bowels. Rae had read of lauded cures in recent texts and was drawn in particular to a scientific study by one of the East India Company's surgeons who had extensive experience with cholera in Madras. This recommended that a particularly noxious hydro-sulphuret of ammonia be added to the enema and went on to predict that within a few years sulphur would be accepted as the cure for cholera in the same way as lemon juice had become universally acknowledged as the cure for scurvy. There were also newspaper reports from North America where physicians likewise claimed success with sulphur treatments and pointed to indisputable evidence that cholera never existed near springs where the water was sulphurated or near volcanoes where the mineral was abundant.

Exotic as some acclaimed remedies were, neither Rae nor Allen was convinced that the different outcomes in cholera cases depended on which treatment was given. Rae had worked throughout the 1832 epidemic. His impression was that this time the disease had returned in a more virulent form and was proving more rapidly fatal. 'However, anything is worthy of trial,' he suggested. 'I fear we shall yet have too many instances of testing the efficacy of sulphur as well as other remedies – all probably equally futile.' It was extremely difficult to judge the severity of a cholera attack. A marine brought in on 23 July with abdominal cramps seemed to respond well to the care provided. Rae had marked him down as on the long road to recovery: food and water were being retained and the patient free from pain and very comfortable. 'But in a few minutes,' Rae noted with astonishment, 'he was found to be moribund.'[8] The secret, if there was one, Rae and Allen agreed, lay in being able to tend to sufferers at the onset of the disease and then operating a strict routine of constant nursing.

Gaining rapid access to cholera victims, however, proved an unsolvable problem. If seamen were struck down in their houses the time taken to diagnose and send them to the Royal Naval Hospital might prove too long. Similarly with men aboard the ships at anchor, where the surgeon might undertake a treatment for diarrhoea or choleraic diarrhoea and only when too late discover that Asiatic cholera had taken hold. Seamen were thus often admitted to the wards when all hope had gone, which was both an unnecessary loss of life and an unfair reflection on the hospital's effectiveness. There was, though, one source of entry where Rae had some influence. Many cholera victims were marines who lived in the nearby barracks. The Royal Marine barracks had its own infirmary, but serious cases of injury or illness were never treated there and regulations required a prompt transfer to the Royal Naval Hospital of all life-threatening ailments. Throughout July 1849 the barracks was mercifully free of cholera and all the marines who succumbed lived out in one of the towns. But by 10 August there had been at least seven severe cases diagnosed in the marine barracks, most of whom had died on transfer to the hospital. Rae had wanted to inspect sanitary conditions inside the barracks earlier, but only this sudden outbreak had persuaded the Port Admiral to authorise a visit. This gave Rae the opportunity to investigate not only whether the barracks themselves were kept in a proper state of cleanliness but also the efficiency of the surgeon and his assistant there in diagnosing and moving infected men. Rae conceded afterwards that all at the barracks seemed to be in order. He would leave no stone unturned, though, to ensure that the hospital would not be found wanting in the present crisis and that Nicolas would never have just cause to criticise his medical management.

By 12 August Rae had treated fifty-seven cholera patients in the wards with a further thirty-three tended for choleraic diarrhoea. He had already lost sixteen cases and still had twenty-three under treatment, some of whom were unlikely to recover. The Royal Naval Hospital was now experiencing the epidemic with the same force as it had earlier struck the local authorities. On 9 August the cholera wards had admitted eighteen patients, five of whom died within hours. But Rae was not one for panic even though his strict regime of round-the-clock nursing was under considerable pressure. 'We are doing all we can,' he noted, 'have wards and beds constantly in readiness and also nurses at hand so that not a moment may be lost.'[9] The hospital's nurses were, in fact, little more than ward orderlies and Rae was careful to keep up their spirits. Their work was livened twice daily by the ounce of brandy which he doled out to every man. He was full of praise for the young assistant-surgeons who watched over the victims day and night, and for Allen, whose steadfastness relieved so much of the burden from his own shoulders. With only a small medical staff he was operating one ward for the serious Asiatic cholera cases and two others for those who showed premonitory symptoms – in addition, of course, to the normal medical and surgical demands placed on the hospital. The only comforting fact was that no cholera had yet been diagnosed inside the institution; every case had been admitted either from the marine barracks or from the towns.

Although Rae had found nothing amiss when he toured the marine barracks on 10 August, he continued to worry about it as a source of disease. In London, however, Burnett already knew a great deal about the barracks and its infirmary and had in fact been using it, rather than the Royal Naval Hospital, to investigate cholera since the start of the epidemic. The surgeon at the barracks was Andrew Millar, who reported directly to Burnett and for whose skill and intelligence the latter had a high regard. Millar was helped by William Kay, an outstanding twenty-seven-year-old assistant-surgeon, already seven years in the Navy, to whom Burnett later referred as 'in every respect a *most superior* and talented officer. Few are equal to him in the service'.[10] Millar and Kay not only knew their barracks, but they knew all the haunts where marines lived, and were accustomed to visiting the men and their families. As late as mid-July Millar was certain that no marine had yet contracted cholera, though the battalion took every precaution. Night passes from the barracks were curtailed and daily reporting on the sanitary arrangements in the quarters occupied by married men was introduced.

On 21 July Burnett specifically requested Kay to visit the areas of East Stonehouse where cholera was spreading; by this time there had been a few deaths among the marines and their families, some of whom had been tended by Millar and others by private practitioners. Kay identified one potential source of the disease straight away at the rear of the barracks and on the quayside where the local dock company had allowed refuse to pile up. Millar impressed the urgency of this on the commanding officer of marines in Plymouth, who at once gained approval from London for legal action against the dock company through the Admiralty solicitor. Kay went out to report again ten days later. The state of the housing and the dirt in the streets, he concluded, would explain why not only cholera but fever, scrofula, rheumatism and other ailments were so prevalent among the population. Kay examined the defective drainage which contributed to the state of the courts where so many of the marines lived and drew attention to some of the worst deposits of dirt which, though not immediately visible, lay within twenty feet of each of the two main entrances to the barracks. Kay was not only a medic of remarkable perception and with real understanding of public health issues, Millar told Burnett, but he had also built up a unique knowledge of the backstreets in many parts of Plymouth and East Stonehouse and identified nuisances unlikely to be discovered by officers of their Boards of Health.

Millar's enthusiasm for Kay's public health studies did not, of course, mean that the infirmary could afford his absence and on 30 July Millar asked Burnett for an additional assistant to help with the cholera cases. By now both he and Kay were quite exhausted. Kay's findings, though, did explain to Millar's satisfaction why the poor rate in East Stonehouse was always so high. Not only was it a parish with fewer wealthy residents to pay the rate than Plymouth, but many of its poorer inhabitants were also chronically ill and therefore unable to support themselves. 'Inability to labour from impaired health is well known to attend persons living amidst impurities of so gross a nature as those described,' Millar reflected. The East Stonehouse Guardians 'would confer the greatest boon on the inhabitants by improving the health of all classes and materially lessening the tax of the poor rate.'[11] Burnett, however, was not interested in a lecture on political economy, being preoccupied by this time with two more pressing concerns: first, devising further tests for his own chloride of zinc following Bowden's experiment at Noss and second with the need to find extra surgeons and assistants from the half-pay list with which to meet not only Millar's but also similar calls for assistance on account of cholera from other naval institutions.

With respect to the chloride, even while Bowden had been in Noss Burnett had directed that the Royal Naval Hospital should also monitor its effectiveness when treating cholera cases. On 16 July he ordered extensive use in the wards, whereby it was to be sprinkled on the floors, over bedding and on to any discharges from patients. Bodies of the dead were to be sponged with the fluid before being removed wrapped in sheets previously soaked therein. Labourers in the mortuary were likewise to wash their hands and faces with it before handling corpses. The clothing and bedding of all cholera patients were also to be immersed in the solution for forty-eight hours before washing. At the Royal Marine Infirmary too Millar was told to use it freely in order to keep the barracks clean; he applied it similarly to the decks and interior of HMS *Nemesis*, which had been sent as a refuge for healthy marines and their families.

While the medical staff supervised such use within the hospital and infirmary, Nicolas ensured that chloride of zinc was employed as widely as possible by the civic authorities. He recommended it to the Guardians of East Stonehouse and at a meeting with Beer he urged the Plymouth Board of Health to place an order for a supply to be sent down from London. On 22 July he even began to advise Burnett on how best to sell the product: Burnett's agent would do well to form a business link with a druggist in Plymouth through whom orders could be placed. 'I have caused its abundant use here,' he boasted to Burnett. Although it was inappropriate for a senior naval officer holding his position to make or to recommend any particular contact for distributing the solution, his immediate reference to 'Beer, the chemist from East Street, Plymouth' could not possibly have evaded Burnett's notice.[12]

Nicolas had no doubt that the chloride was effective in limiting the epidemic and he believed that he could demonstrate this by the fact that not one person who had worked in the naval hospital's cholera wards had contracted the disease. 'I attribute this *principally*, if not *wholly*, to the free use of the chloride of zinc,' he asserted. Nor was that all. When out in the town with Milroy, McClure had also used the solution in the dwellings of the poor where 'pestilential effluvia speedily disappeared '*as if by magic*.'[13] Burnett was naturally intrigued but, of course, realised that simply handing out his fluid from Admiralty supplies and then claiming that Plymouth was healthier did not constitute cause and effect and he discouraged Nicolas from dispensing his patented chemical gratis to the local authorities. The chance to conduct another controlled trial, however, arose unexpectedly at the beginning of August 1849 after the General Board of Health suddenly ordered Milroy to abandon his study of cholera in the naval towns and to proceed into Cornwall, thereby making available for other work much of the time which McClure had previously devoted to acting as Milroy's voluntary assistant.

Milroy was sent to deal with an emergency in Mevagissey, from where reports reached London that half of its 2,310 panic-stricken inhabitants had fled as cholera took a severe toll. Having lost the services of its one medical practitioner, and about to lose those of another as the burden of tending to the sick became too great, the chairman of the Union Guardians rode to Plymouth for help and was allowed to employ temporarily one of the town's district surgeons. Milroy arrived at the end of July and found Mevagissey so depleted that members of its Board of Health were themselves obliged to carry coffins to the graves. Milroy succeeded in organising medical provision, removing many nuisances and evacuating the healthy to tents outside the village, although not before 126 cholera deaths had been recorded and not without a generous provision of 112lbs of Burnett's fluid which Nicolas had allowed him to take from the Royal Naval Hospital. Burnett turned a blind eye to that; by the time he found out he was already issuing large amounts of it to McClure along with directions on how to use it in a new trial in some of the worst parts of Plymouth.

With Milroy gone, McClure was delighted to have a further chance to engage in public health work outside the naval hospital. As directed by Burnett, he selected squalid areas off Stonehouse Lane where cholera was most rampant and then applied the chloride 'not only in the houses but also in a number of foul drains, cesspools etc'. All this he recorded carefully, he assured Burnett, 'in order that I might have an opportunity of testing its efficacy as a purifying agent'.[14] McClure's experiment lasted for about two weeks, his supply of the solution being exhausted by 15 August. In that time he encountered stinking rooms, cellars and drains where the chloride, used as a disinfecting agent, had removed foul odours and purified the air for the benefit of all those who lived crammed into the surrounding courts and alleys. McClure went further in his efforts to establish medical results. He found a multi-room house with fifty-two inhabitants where cholera had struck several times. Most rooms were liberally sprinkled with the fluid, but in four rooms the inhabitants refused the application. Contrasting the different rooms, in those sprinkled no cholera cases had since arisen, whereas in the other four rooms the disease still existed and some fatalities had occurred. Two houses immediately opposite had likewise been thoroughly sprayed and experienced no cholera cases, whereas in houses all around them the disease was raging. This, McClure was convinced, constituted the scientific proof Burnett had hoped for from Bowden's work at Noss.

To support his thesis McClure also produced medical testimony from two district surgeons whom he had included in his experiment. Fox wrote from five fields that in his experience both there, in his medical district and aboard a hulk where he had also attended cholera patients, Burnett's fluid was by far the most effective disinfecting agent. John Benbow, from the second district of the Plymouth Board of Health, wrote not only of its superior disinfecting qualities but, like McClure, cited a property where he had used it after choleraic diarrhoea cases had been diagnosed but where the disease had since subsided and the remaining residents enjoyed good health. 'The fluid was used according to your directions,' Benbow assured McClure on 11 August, and the results 'much to my surprise and delight.'[15] McClure's results and those of his medical colleagues in the town were passed on to the Board of Admiralty and to the General Board of Health. One immediate outcome was that Fox and Prance had been so impressed with the trial at the cholera hospital that 'on their recommendation the Plymouth Board of Health have ordered a large supply from London for the use of that establishment'.[16] When settling the Board's account with a banker's order, its deputy chairman added that wherever in Plymouth the chemical had been freely used cholera had not reappeared, whereas in areas where its application had been constrained the disease had broken out a second time.[17] This was all excellent news for Burnett. Not only had McClure gathered expert testimony but, crucially, he seemed to have been able to test the value of the solution against controls in a crowded urban environment the likes of which had never been available to Bowden at Noss. Whether this was ultimately proof or not, in August 1849 McClure had succeeded in taking the process of experimentation an important step on. Furthermore, he had done so while clearly earning admiration from those with whom he had worked. Benbow was profuse in his thanks for the help he had received, which, he assured McClure, the poor of Plymouth greatly appreciated. McClure naturally ensured that such flattering observations quickly found their way to London, where Burnett in turn passed them on to the General Board of Health. It was a wonderful commendation for the naval medical service, in addition to which the evidence amassed, as with the material which Bowden had assembled from Noss, could all be used in future advertisement for the chloride. McClure's standing as an assistant-surgeon of exceptional promise could scarcely have been higher.

While arranging for McClure to begin his trial Burnett had also to meet the urgent appeals for assistance arriving from naval hospitals and infirmaries. Millar's case for an additional surgeon was clear cut and promptly met; predictably this encouraged a similar request for cholera cover from the Royal Naval Hospital where Nicolas warned Burnett that there appeared to be no end to cases among the marines and that Rae and his colleagues were almost worn out with round-the-clock attention to these patients. But that was not all. Nicolas needed more labourers and washerwomen, the former to dig graves and to make more hair beds and the latter to clean thoroughly all the linen of cholera patients; in the emergency he had already hired two extra of each and now sought the Admiralty's permission further to increase his staff during the epidemic. Burnett had to accept that the hospital could no longer function with its existing staff and selected three officers from the half-pay list to proceed there at once. Richard Mason, a full surgeon since 1844, was to assist Rae and Allen by taking charge of the cholera wards while Augustus Preston and William Gruggen were sent as additional assistant-surgeons. Three further surgeons on half pay resident in Plymouth were ordered to be ready to serve on ships and in naval establishments as the Port Admiral might decide. In the circumstances the Board of Admiralty also allowed Nicolas the auxiliaries he had requested.

The Royal Naval Hospital and the Marine Infirmary, however, were not the only medical institutions in the service to find their resources stretched by an influx of cholera patients, and by the beginning of August 1849 and for weeks to come Burnett was distracted from the problems in Plymouth by his search for extra staff to help out at Chatham, Greenwich and Portsmouth. Chatham was initially the worst affected because the cholera epidemic was exacerbated by a simultaneous outbreak of smallpox. On 15 August Thomas Stratton was sent to the Melville hospital as an additional surgeon with an assistant also provided a few days later. Stratton arrived as the hospital had forty-one cholera cases under care and was clearly in a state of disarray. The Melville's regular staff were overwhelmed trying to run four wards for cholera patients day and night while tending to a further seven smallpox victims in an isolation unit made by converting the operating theatre. Meanwhile the basement was used for the gonorrhoea and other cases on the hospital's books, even though it was quite unequipped for the task. At Burnett's urging, the Board of Admiralty sanctioned the cost of covering the damp stone basement floors with wooden planking and fitting water closets. The Melville's register listed 234 inmates on 23 August – the largest number since it had opened in 1828. At the corresponding date in 1848 there had been only 130. Nevertheless, cholera was never so severe in Chatham as in Plymouth and from a population of 60,000 Chatham and its neighbourhood had recorded only forty-nine deaths by late August. The Gillingham, Rochester and Strood districts recorded together a further 164 cholera deaths by mid-September, but by then the epidemic had largely run its course in the Medway towns.[18]

In so far as any other naval establishment had to cope with cholera in a way at all comparable to those at Plymouth or Chatham it was the infirmary at Greenwich which served the pensioners of the Hospital and the 900 boys of the naval schools. The Greenwich Hospital Foundation was independent of Burnett's department at the Admiralty; nevertheless he was asked to recommend an extra surgeon for service there in September 1849 when cholera suddenly spread through the institution at an alarming rate. A dozen of the old pensioners had died by 11 September and on the previous day alone twenty-four schoolboys had been diagnosed. A day later thirty-three boys were in the infirmary and the danger was considered so great that a hulk was ordered to stand by for an evacuation.[19] The Greenwich Hospital eventually lost thirty-two from among the seventy-seven old men afflicted, although – remarkably – all the schoolboys survived. Portsmouth required two assistant-surgeons to be found from Burnett's diminishing half-pay list; one was assigned to the Marine Infirmary and another to the *Victory* for cholera duty among convicts. The Haslar, however, was spared the same wave of admissions which put Rae and his staff under such pressure at East Stonehouse.[20]

Indeed, with no help yet arrived, so hopelessly overburdened was Rae with the number of cholera admissions to the Royal Naval Hospital that his treatments were becoming increasingly desperate. His report to Burnett on two cases lost on 14 August revealed the crude use of mechanical pressure, by way of a bung, in forlorn attempts to keep fluid in the body. Beforehand he had administered the usual calomel, sesquicarbonate of ammonia and brandy and then injected sulphate of zinc and laudanum directly into the large intestine in the hope of quelling muscular spasms. Despite his efforts to speed up transfers from the Marine Infirmary it remained generally true that the hospital received disproportionately high numbers of serious cases too advanced for effective treatment: cases were being brought in when the pulse was scarcely perceptible. He had expected some easing in the number of fresh cases in the three towns, but this had not occurred nor was there any sign of respite. Eighteen cholera deaths were recorded in Plymouth on 12 August with a further seven in East Stonehouse and more in Devonport. 'Thank God I am well,' Rae exclaimed in response, 'but I do not get over my morning visit until after twelve and then have some headache from thought and anxiety.'[21]

Mason and the two assistant-surgeons arrived on 13 and 14 August and immediately enabled Rae to transform his medical regime. Rae and Allen thereafter devoted their attention to regular illnesses and surgery, visiting the cholera wards but twice daily in order to ensure that the routine and treatments prescribed were being followed. Mason also took charge of the extra nurses allowed by the Admiralty and organised a twenty-four-hour relay for the constant supervision of helpless patients. Cholera cases were never left without a surgeon or assistant on duty. The pressure on Rae also eased in mid-August, when the Admiralty ordered that a cholera hospital should be set up inside the dockyard at Devonport. This had to be equipped with stores of sheets, mattresses and clothing from the Royal Naval Hospital, but it possessed all the facilities necessary to care for seamen and artisans who worked in the yard at every stage of the illness, thereby ending Rae's admissions from this quarter. The dockyard surgeon and his assistant, like Millar and Kay at the Royal Marine Infirmary, were also responsible for the care of men and their families in their homes and were consequently closely in touch with the spread of cholera in the vicinity. The dockyard alone had reported twenty-one cholera deaths by 24 August, rising to thirty-eight by the end of the following month. When Rae wrote with considerable relief, therefore, on 20 August that the epidemic seemed to be abating, it was difficult to judge initially whether there were really fewer cases or whether the cases were simply being treated elsewhere. It was none the less a fact that there had been no cholera diagnosed among the marines for four days and no admissions to the hospital since 18 August. Nineteen cholera patients were discharged cured on 21 August. This was the first piece of good news that Rae had sent to London since the epidemic began. Outside the hospital walls, though, and where the local Boards of Health were in charge, things had gone from bad to worse.

CHAPTER 8

Litigation, the Press and the Navy

As Rae struggled to maintain efficient working at the Royal Naval Hospital, in the towns around it the epidemic was clearly spreading. In Plymouth the weekly figures for 2 August indicated 162 cases, with twenty-seven deaths. Those published on 9 August revealed 262 cases, with twenty-eight deaths; those of 16 August 827 cases, with eighty-four deaths and those of 23 August 347 cases, with seventy-five deaths. Yet the authorities there remained largely above the criticism which continued to be directed at the Guardians of East Stonehouse for having allowed cholera to run out of control. In fact, Latimer praised Plymouth's magistrates for the promptness with which they had dealt with complaints about public health nuisances, while the mayor was commended for his decisive use of the police force to remove all pigs from areas where the disease was at its worst without waiting for 'the tardy and uncertain process required by Act of Parliament'.[1] Furthermore, the five-fields hospital was judged to be coping with the crisis: Fox and Prance had tended no fewer than 240 patients in the first week of August.

The Plymouth authorities were certainly conscious that it was important to be seen to be active. When the town surveyor reported an overflow of some drains to the Improvement Commissioners on 7 August the decision to invite tenders was not only duly minuted by the management committee but, for the benefit of the General Board of Health, Milroy was invited to witness the earnest discussion on the importance of efficient drainage which ensued.[2] The Plymouth Guardians showed themselves equally astute by their handling of the press. When Beer and Morrish went out to inspect the backstreets in some of the poorest areas on 8 August they made sure that a journalist accompanied them. Seeing for himself the dilapidated, ill-drained, ill-ventilated and overcrowded housing in which the poor lived, and the dirt which so characterised their interiors, the writer was moved to applaud the efforts of men who risked their own health tending to the public good. Blame should be apportioned to the inhabitants; had the Plymouth Board of Health not taken matters so seriously things could only be worse.

Trailing around the town with their well-chosen reporter in tow, Beer and Morrish naturally elaborated on all that had been done in the face of apparently insuperable barriers to improving the welfare of Plymouth's citizenry. Cholera sufferers were moved to five fields, backstreets slushed with water, pigs were turned loose and their sties demolished and men sent into the worst areas to whitewash the buildings inside and out. 'To Mr. Joseph Beer the town owes a deep debt of gratitude,' the *Journal* obligingly recorded. 'It was he who grappled with the disease at its commencement.' Beer's skill with this medium produced two further points of reassurance for its readership on 9 August, both of which naturally reflected well on the Board of Health. First, the five-fields hospital was adequate and well supplied and no further money was required. There was a widespread rumour that a second cholera hospital was needed to cope with the epidemic. 'This is altogether untrue,' Latimer stated definitively. 'The Board of Health could not see a necessity for such an expense being incurred.'[3] Second, the disease was being broadly confined not only to the poorest classes but even here disproportionately to drunkards. This was revealed as information from a medical source: the extent of illness was, therefore, something for which no public body could legitimately be held accountable.

Although the cholera figures for Plymouth barely improved throughout August, the Board of Health still managed to avoid adverse comment. On 23 August the *Journal* remarked again on the Board's proper precautions and stressed the importance of individual exertions for removing the conditions which caused disease. The owners of properties were now chastised for their slowness in cleaning up land and buildings adjacent to inhabited areas. Personal hygiene, diet and bodily exercise continued to be cited as the best safeguards against infection, without which the valiant efforts of the Board of Health would prove useless. The Board should not have needed recourse to law in so many instances: its work for the public good had encountered too many obstacles from self-interest and indifferent residents. This was a notable public endorsement of the Board's endeavours for which the authorities in Devonport and especially in East Stonehouse would have been profoundly grateful.

Devonport never received the same press coverage as did Plymouth and East Stonehouse. Cholera came later to Devonport and the authorities collected and released less information. By the beginning of August, though, cholera was well established in the town and the Board of Health there was holding daily meetings. Several orders for the removal of nuisances had been served and a temporary hospital and house of refuge were being erected on land owned by the Board of Ordnance. Up to 8 August a total of 127 persons had died from cholera in Devonport, most of them during the last week. This included ten in the workhouse, from where the children were all immediately evacuated.[4] A further 125 died in the week up to 15 August and 129 in the week to 22 August. These were much higher rates of fatality than for Plymouth, yet again the press seemed reluctant to criticise the local authority, later judging that the Devonport Board of Health had adopted all the proper precautionary measures. It was never vouchsafed, however, what these measures were other than that the Board had accepted the material help which the Admiralty had been quick to make available. Nicolas lent twelve iron bedsteads from the Royal Naval Hospital in order to help set up the Devonport Board's cholera hospital on 8 August while the Admiralty agreed to provide a hulk containing 300 hammocks for the use of convalescent patients two weeks later. Even so, it was 10 September before the Devonport cholera hospital, with its two medical staff, was fully operational. In the final week of August and first week of September cholera deaths in Devonport were eighty-one and forty-five respectively while the comparable totals in Plymouth were fifty and thirty-eight – and this when the overall numbers of cases diagnosed were much the same.

To the Guardians of East Stonehouse, therefore, it seemed most unfair that while their counterparts in Plymouth were reported so favourably, and those in Devonport so little, scrutiny of them was so harsh and unrelenting. In August, as before, the reason for that lay largely with Nicolas's activities at the Royal Naval Hospital and the publicity he attracted. The cholera figures for East Stonehouse were never as bad as the criticism heaped on the authorities there suggested. While both the Plymouth and Devonport Boards reported three-figure death totals in the second week of August, that in East Stonehouse recorded only fifteen. In the week ending 22 August, when their death tolls were seventy-five and 129 respectively, the figure in East Stonehouse was only nine. Likewise in the week to 29 August, the twelve deaths in East Stonehouse seemed very few compared to fifty in Plymouth and eighty-one in Devonport and the same remained true into the first week of September when East Stonehouse recorded only six cholera deaths against thirty-eight and forty-five in the other two towns. Admittedly the East Stonehouse authorities had never shown the same initiative in tackling cholera as those in Plymouth and they had certainly done nothing to court the press. Nevertheless events seemed to conspire against them and to expose them to public outcry where they were not really to blame. On 2 August, for instance, the *Journal* made much of the fact that the East Stonehouse Board had received a sharp letter from Chadwick and Southwood-Smith at the General Board of Health which had been critical about the provision of medical officers to tend the poor and the failure to erect a cholera hospital. Yet the Guardians had appointed five practitioners for the poor of East Stonehouse: they had merely neglected to divide the Union into separate districts, assigning a specific doctor to each. As for a hospital, there was simply no land in the Union which any owner would make available or allow to be used without making legal objections on the grounds of danger to adjoining habitations.

All efforts to find a plot proving futile, the Guardians turned to Nicolas, requesting the temporary use of a piece of ground on the eastern side of the naval hospital. Nicolas set aside all his disagreements with the Guardians and promptly agreed. This was also after a deputation had been sent to the Plymouth Board of Health asking if in the circumstances the five-fields hospital might admit some patients from East Stonehouse, which the Plymouth authorities had flatly refused. Likewise in East Stonehouse there was no building suitable as a house of refuge for the healthy until Nicolas again obliged by allowing the use of a naval prison. The press seemed interested only in the removal of visible or nasal nuisances – work where the East Stonehouse Board was at its weakest but which the death rates should have indicated made very little difference either to the severity of the disease or to the rate of mortality. Writing scathingly, but with a highly selective focus, on 9 August the *Journal* was adamant that in the war against nuisances the authorities in East Stonehouse 'appear not yet to have learnt what a nuisance is'.[5]

Behind this slowness to act in East Stonehouse lay, Latimer asserted, a refusal to spend money even in a time of crisis. This was also Nicolas's view as he continued his campaign both in the press and by litigation to clean up the environs of the Royal Naval Hospital. He reported to Burnett on 9 August that despite the enquiry at the Queen's Arms on 31 July nothing had happened about the filth piled up at dung wharf which, following some further deaths close by, he was more certain than ever represented a threat to residents, those who passed by on the water and to patients inside the hospital. The local Board of Health had legal powers to act, he stated, 'but appear wilfully blind to the existence of those flagrant abuses and still continue so'. 'I earnestly trust that the General Board of Health, or the Poor Law Commissioners, will interfere to make the Board of Health of Stonehouse do its duty,' he continued pessimistically, 'for unless the *law* will *force* these persons to act in these cases I fear that nothing will be done.'[6] But his criticism displayed the same refusal to examine the statistics carefully as did the *Journal's* reporting. Nicolas was quick to point out that since cholera was first diagnosed in East Stonehouse on 13 July about sixty victims had succumbed, but less willing to acknowledge that the seventy or so further deaths around Stonehouse Lane, often equally close to the hospital, had occurred within the boundaries of the Plymouth Board of Health.

The East Stonehouse Guardians defended themselves as best they could. On 6 August they published a response to the General Board of Health's criticisms, in which they pointed out that they had formed a local Board of Health to sit daily as soon as cholera had appeared, made medicines and medical aid available to the poor of the parish by the appointment of five practitioners and, after much difficulty, found sites for a cholera hospital and a house of refuge. 'The remarks made by the Press, imputing to them neglect, are without foundation,' the Guardians assured the General Board of Health.[7] True to form, neither the press nor the Navy was convinced. Nicolas revelled in the publicity which his public health campaign provided and had no intention whatever of dropping his litigation.

The Admiralty's suit regarding the deposit at dung wharf was heard at the Petty Sessions in East Stonehouse on 7 August. Eastlake opened the proceedings by listing the failings of the four contractors who operated there to clear the offensive dangers to health and life from the quay; he then went on to allege that some of the Guardians, even after a visit, had refused to acknowledge the nuisance and, contrary to medical opinion, had ordered only a very limited remonstrance against one of the contractors. Nicolas was immediately called to give evidence. He described the offensive atmosphere which wafted across the neighbourhood and into the hospital and he railed at the manner in which the authorities had ignored his thirty letters of complaint. 'These nuisances were as glaring as the sun at noon,' Nicolas insisted, and by the consent of all medical men who knew the area were likely responsible for a dozen or so deaths. Turning to all present, Nicolas declared that his great efforts in this matter sprang from a longing to do justice for the poor. It was, he concluded theatrically, 'a most shameful thing that the lives of the twelve people should have been thrown away.'

McClure was then summoned and duly corroborated his chief's opinions; the state of the quay had not improved in over three weeks. 'It is complained of bitterly by the poor people living about there,' he added, 'but they can get no redress.' The Admiralty solicitor's tactics were plain enough: the Navy would put itself forward as the champion of those too distressed to help themselves. As naval officers and servants of the Crown they would take an interest in the public good when the proper authorities had so clearly failed in their duty. It was a clever approach and one which, given the heightened public alarm about health across the town, was difficult for the Guardians to counter.

Between them, Nicolas and Latimer turned the hearing into a political spectacle. After all the evidence had been heard Nicolas returned to address the assembly, exposing repeated promises by the contractors to remove night soil, offal and pigs from the quay as worthless, stating that he had offered to have the quay cleared by naval labourers and then demanding that notices be served upon the four operators. This was all fully printed in the *Journal*, as was Nicolas's story to the court that he had interrupted his dinner one evening, for such was his concern for the poor, in order to get off his urgent despatch to the Board of Ordnance requesting the use of government land for the

East Stonehouse cholera hospital and of the prison for the house of refuge. After such a performance the Bench gave the worst of the contractors forty-eight hours to remove his dung or else his portion of the quay would be cleaned up for him by the public authorities and a bill presented. Latimer reported all this in a triumphant tone. Nicolas was hailed as a gallant officer crusading against official lethargy and private interest. 'It would have been supposed that a gentleman of energy and unusual determination like Captain Nicolas, occupying the post of Superintendent of the Royal Naval Hospital, would have found no difficulty in getting a nuisance removed that is said to have caused the death of about a dozen people,' Latimer noted sarcastically. 'But no; he possessed no power over the stingy habits of this immovable Board.'

Whatever its failings in matters of public health may have been, the East Stonehouse Board undoubtedly demonstrated its utter incompetence in the realm of public relations and almost certainly made matters worse for itself by not being represented at the Petty Sessions, thereby apparently confirming its indifference to public sentiment. This was an affront not only to the population of East Stonehouse, the *Journal* declared, but to all those who lived in Plymouth and Devonport too. 'The authorities of one of these towns cannot permit a wrong of this kind without the neighbourhood suffering in common and to a like extent with themselves.'[8] Adopting now the same line as Eastlake had taken at the hearing, Latimer announced that his paper was compelled to speak out on behalf of those who otherwise would have no voice. If the wealthy and powerful could not gain for themselves a purer air and better environment then what hope could there be for the poor?

The judgment given on 7 August and the adverse publicity which accompanied it forced the East Stonehouse Board of Health to support the Admiralty's solicitor in issuing summonses for nuisance removal against the other contractors at dung wharf. These further actions were heard in a crowded Plymouth town hall a week later. Nicolas and McClure were there again; both by now were local heroes. Nicolas and Eastlake were not convinced that the East Stonehouse Guardians had experienced a sufficient change of heart and the latter's address to the citizenry present on this occasion was blatantly calculated to exploit parochial divisions and ill feeling. 'The Stonehouse Board of Guardians had charged upon the Plymouth people the introduction of the cholera into their town,' Eastlake asserted. 'They had done very little either to prevent its continuance or to get rid of it.' This time the Guardians were represented in court and one of them leapt up to say that Eastlake should not proceed in this way. Eastlake retorted that he spoke advisedly, to which came the veiled threat that 'you had better not complain against the Board of Guardians'. The two magistrates conducting the hearing restored decorum by announcing that the current action was against contractors, not Guardians, and that any charge against the latter should take another form. For the moment, though, Eastlake could call witnesses to the Board's inaction in the past.

McClure, inhabitants of the parish and a doctor who practised there all gave evidence to the effect that there had been no improvement in sanitation in East Stonehouse since cholera began. McClure then broadened his testimony and spoke out on a fundamental point of public health. He did not just want the deposits of manure on the quayside cleaned up for the current epidemic: for the sake of the health of the town, he advised boldly, future accumulations should also be prevented. To the delight of those packed into the town hall, Eastlake and McClure had transformed a modest legal action into a platform for the expression of deeply felt public concern.

'You cannot have stronger evidence. It must be removed,' the magistrates ruled. Furthermore, piling up soil on the quayside should no longer be permitted. 'The Court did not consider further evidence necessary.' It was a great compliment to McClure, but in setting a forty-eight hour deadline the economic problems which could arise when enforcing public health legislation were also revealed. 'What am I to do?' one of the contractors pleaded. 'It is my living altogether.' For the people who made a precarious and unattractive living scavenging, gathering the night soil of the towns, feeding pigs and collecting offal from slaughterhouses in order to sell it for agricultural benefit, such an order effectively put them out of work and risked throwing them on to poor relief. It was not therefore surprising that Boards of Guardians were often reluctant to begin legal proceedings against them. 'What shall I do with my horse and cart?' the contractor continued. In any case: 'there are others who offend as well as me'. As to the deposit at dung wharf, 'if the gentlemen wish to make me an offer I will take it in the country'. But the forty-eight hour notice came, of course, with no offer of payment. Other offenders would be treated in the same way, the magistrates declared, and if the material was not moved, or if more was allowed to accumulate, then 'the Guardians will bring you up again immediately. There is so much sickness in various parts of Stonehouse that if this should occur again there will be no delay in prosecuting you.' Addressing the town hall crowd when judgment was concluded on all the contractors, the magistrates left no doubt about their sympathies. 'A man said what was he to do with his horse and cart, but what had the Bench got to do with that?' one enquired rhetorically. Some family livelihoods would suffer; nevertheless, with disease rampant across the country, 'the health of the parish is not to be trifled with, and it requires extraordinary measures to preserve the health of the town'. All were keen, it appeared, to jump on to the bandwagon which Nicolas and Latimer had started to roll.

So enamoured had Nicolas become of his new-found public role and so enthusiastic about health reform that the Navy's involvement in litigation went further than just getting orders against the filth on the quayside which affected its own hospital. In his work with Milroy and local doctors McClure had discovered other nuisances which blighted people's lives and which both he and Nicolas were determined to see removed. The worst of these was taken up by Eastlake and formed an action against an East Stonehouse butcher and slaughterer whose premises were repeatedly found to be awash with blood and layers of decomposing matter. This case was heard in the town hall on 14 August, where McClure paraded as the leading witness. It was manna for the *Journal* too. 'This case developed a few of the secrets of pig feeding,' it advertised to the consuming public, 'and it appeared to be listened to with peculiar interest by the eaters of pork sausages.' McClure was backed up by an East Stonehouse practitioner and their evidence was sufficient to persuade the Bench that the problem had to be addressed. It was a slightly awkward case for the Admiralty to bring; the butcher was quick to point out in his defence that troops were supplied from his premises. In consequence, the number of animals killed there was very large but care was taken to prevent excessive accumulations of waste product. When pressed as to how this was done, however, it transpired that live pigs were kept in the slaughterhouse in order to eat up the offal spilt from those newly butchered. 'Those animals are the only means I have of making the place more clean,' the hapless butcher implored the magistrates, at which point the town hall resounded with laughter and derision and the Bench ordered the immediate removal of both the pigs and the disgusting debris of the abattoir, the evil odour of which was held to have contributed in all likelihood to as many as seventeen cholera deaths.[9]

Bad as relations between the civil and naval authorities in East Stonehouse had undoubtedly become by mid-August 1849, Nicolas was still willing to provide whatever material help he could. On 12 August the Guardians were obliged to swallow their pride and beg the loan of a few iron bedsteads for the use of families in the house of refuge. The Devonport Board of Health already had a dozen such beds on loan and Nicolas could hardly refuse the East Stonehouse Guardians what he had granted others or, indeed, when he had constantly criticised them for inadequate provision. His help for the East Stonehouse authorities, however, was more grudgingly given. Its Board of Health had guaranteed to return everything in proper order; nevertheless, 'I have directed that the *oldest* articles be selected for this loan,' he wrote to Burnett.[10] Two days later the East Stonehouse Guardians were back with another request: their cholera hospital had no tanks for water storage. Nicolas arranged a loan of two from dockyard stores.[11]

Yet even with Nicolas finding the land and supplying hardware, the Guardians still seemed unable to erect a basic hospital facility. By 21 August it remained unfinished, the roof of the tent being still open along the seams and there being no furniture other than the few beds lent from the Royal Naval Hospital. This was in clear breach of the directions issued by the General Board of Health, Latimer reminded the population, and it typified the indifference of the East Stonehouse authorities, who had effectively relied upon the individual efforts of the Captain-Superintendent of the naval hospital to investigate, identify and bring legal actions to remove hazards to public health. Bungling over the cholera hospital proved to be the final straw. This fiasco had cost many lives and Latimer was determined to expose the matter in all its detail. For the Guardians it did indeed make depressing reading.

When the Plymouth Board of Health put up the five-fields hospital in mid-July 1849 the timetable between the initial decision and the first patients admitted to a structure a hundred feet long by thirty feet broad and with gas and water laid was a mere four days. By contrast, the East Stonehouse Board took eight days simply to get tenders for a ninety-four feet by twenty-seven feet construction, having first engaged an architect to plan a wooden structure 'that any man of common sense might have chalked out on a deal board in half an hour'. Then the plan had to be altered, the original having tastelessly provided for a dead house to adjoin the end of the hospital. When advertising the work the East Stonehouse Board sought only to keep costs to a minimum, the *Journal* charged: 'they advertised for the *lowest* tender in a work of emergency – a work of life and death like this'. Worse still, the cheapest contractor was from out of town and had to be granted a fortnight in which to complete the task. 'Is another word necessary?' Latimer asked furiously. The final and most damning judgment on the edifice was that its facilities were so bad that some doctors refused to send patients to it. Yet still the only response from the East Stonehouse authorities to any criticism were terse statements that accusations of neglect were without foundation. 'We have not gone out of our way to condemn the acts of a public body without a great necessity,' the *Journal* concluded sanctimoniously. However, 'the Press in its independence would be disgraced if it did not do its duty at such a time'.[12]

Impervious as the East Stonehouse Guardians remained to criticism, it was more difficult to fend off the General Board of Health with simple denials of shortcomings. The letter from London at the end of July had not only required a cholera hospital and house of refuge to be provided and medical officers to be appointed, but had also stipulated the need for daily visits among the habitations of the poor and a constant monitoring of the symptoms associated with the early stages of cholera. The General Board had urged too that the Guardians provide depots for dispensing medicines to the poor at all hours of the day and night. By late August there were still no signs that any systematic visitations had been organised or any dispensaries established. Writing to the Poor Law Board on 12 August, Rodd sought to excuse the dilatory response of the Guardians by the fact that he had been a victim of severe choleraic diarrhoea and unable therefore to fulfil his duties as clerk as he would have wished. Before he was struck down, however, he had arranged notices for the removal of nuisances to be posted throughout East Stonehouse from mid-July onwards and had made plain to the inhabitants that the local Board of Health once constituted did have statutory powers for inspection and remedy.

But there was more to the shortcomings of the East Stonehouse Board of Health than illness. Having observed its clerk at work for some time, Gulson noted that Rodd was 'of a very sensitive and nervous temperament and he feels keenly where others would take little notice'.[13] These personal characteristics, in fact, impaired the Board's work, since Rodd did not think it fair that he should be expected automatically to act as clerk for this body when his duties were confined to the work of the Board of Guardians. Had it simply involved meeting under another name and without extra work, as indeed was the case for many of the elected Guardians, then Rodd might not have objected so much. But once the cholera epidemic reached East Stonehouse and the Board of Health began its daily meetings after 13 July, Rodd found himself immersed in a routine which both weakened his health and exploited his, albeit modest, sense of public duty. With only his son to help him, Rodd was now 'attending nightly meetings from 7 o'clock p.m. till half past 9 or 10 o'clock.' 'Every night making returns daily to the Board of Health and the public authorities in this town and neighbourhood,' he continued, 'keeping the minutes of all proceedings, giving many notices in cases of nuisance and copies thereof, and generally carrying out all orders of the Board.'[14] Rodd referred his grievance to the Poor Law Board in London, which ruled that a clerk to Union Guardians was required to attend those Guardians in all their business, even when constituted as a Board of Health. At a future date the Guardians might care to acknowledge Rodd's additional duties with a gratuity but that was a matter between the Guardians and their clerk. This ruling merely emphasised how much implementation of parliamentary legislation depended on the energy and initiative of public-spirited individuals. It seemed that in a time of crisis the East Stonehouse Union had not produced men of enterprise and dedication from among its Guardians such as Beer and Morrish had proved themselves to be in neighbouring Plymouth.

Wranglings between the East Stonehouse Guardians and the press lasted throughout August and into September 1849 but the former never managed to cast off the stigma of niggardliness which characterised their handling of the cholera epidemic. When they claimed that the *Journal* had been biased in its reporting of the litigation and of the accusations made against them Latimer was able to refute the allegation by printing letters from Nicolas, Eastlake and McClure, all in support of his paper and vouching for the accuracy of what had been published. Frustrated at the relentless ridicule to which they were subjected, the Guardians then made the gross error of insinuating that they had been 'opposed at every step by the government and other authorities'. Nicolas, not unreasonably, felt that this shot was intended for him and wrote at once to Rodd, pointing out that 'your own official letters to me give the *direct contradiction* to this assertion', threatening thereby to release the copious correspondence between them during the past six weeks. Again the Guardians had to accept defeat. In reply Rodd acknowledged 'the exertions you have made in procuring for them the required supplies for carrying out the regulations and arrangements at the house of refuge and cholera hospital'.[15] In vindication of its own consistent stand against the East Stonehouse authorities and much to Nicolas's personal satisfaction, the *Journal* blazoned this final concession on 30 August. It was the end of a damaging campaign against the Guardians which, though slow to produce any visible improvement in public health provision across the parish, had brought individual abuses and the wider issues which surrounded them into the open and which certainly had seen the standing and competence of those who held public office questioned as never before.

CHAPTER 9

Reaching the People: Controlling the Doctors

PUBLIC HEALTH LEGISLATION in the 1840s was concerned primarily with the creation of new administrative structures and with the legal powers to be conferred upon them; it was largely intended to improve the cleanliness of public places by removing identifiable nuisances to general health. The legislation did not – and of course in many areas could not – lay down particular procedures in the event of epidemics, still less could it specify how the measures undertaken by local authorities might, in practice, reach those for whose benefit they were intended. Official provision and popular usage did not necessarily coincide, although this was by no means always the fault of those bodies responsible for the welfare of the poor. As debates about quarantine restriction and the medical benefits of cholera hospitals indicated, achieving either political or scientific consensus on what might be most appropriate was seldom easy. Even when there was no disagreement, delivery to the needy and gaining their compliance often posed a further set of difficulties. What connected the sick poor with the facilities and organisation set up on their behalf?

Cultural constraints could certainly impede an adequate connection. 'It is too often the case that from false motives of pride, or from terror for which there is no ground, parties who have been taken with the disease refuse to be carried to the hospital,' the *Journal* observed, 'and will rather die in their own close, confined and pestilential dwellings'.[1] Erecting cholera hospitals and houses of refuge conformed with the advice issued to local Boards of Health and in many cases, as at five fields in Plymouth, undoubtedly improved the chances of survival for patients helped to them quickly by friends or family. But the outreach of any hospital was inevitably limited. Finding cholera victims, and thereby sometimes the worst-affected premises in a town from which the disease might spread further, could be a hit-and-miss affair. Street visits by extra parish surgeons and by public-spirited officers from local Guardians or Boards of Health seemed to be an answer but, with scanty personnel available, not knowing exactly where to go and what might lie behind the closed doors of private dwellings made this type of investigation imprecise. It was easy to argue in favour of domestic visits on the grounds that, if detected early, serious cases might sometimes be averted and the spread of cholera thwarted, but during an epidemic time was not on the side of those who undertook such distressing work.[2] It had not succeeded in Edinburgh in 1848, the university's professor of medicine, William Alison, reported grimly: most attacks occurred during the night so that any visit might be too late. Even when victims were discovered, he complained, 'almost all these cases have been mismanaged'.[3]

Sutherland rejected this and remained a firm believer in street visits. His confidence was reinforced by his own experience in Dumfries in December 1848 when he had found it necessary to take charge of the town's public health amid scenes of chaos. Dumfries had 10,000 inhabitants and cholera had raged there since 15 November. By 6 December seventy-eight deaths from among 219 cases had been reported, yet when Sutherland arrived to inspect the work of its Board of Health he found that nothing beyond talking had occurred. 'The regulations of the Board appear to be so much waste paper,' he wrote angrily. Equally deplorable was his discovery that a further forty-seven cholera victims had been buried without their cases even being reported. At once Sutherland instituted dispensaries in the town which would help the poor by day and by night, he organised a house of refuge and he introduced house-to-house visits by resident practitioners and officials. The meeting with the parish Board of Health on 8 December was a stormy affair at which the inspector spoke his mind. 'In all my experience I have met with nothing like this,' he later confided. 'My very spirit is crushed at the want of action of the people.'[4] But his vigour in Dumfries was rewarded and house-to-house visits amid the slums of towns and cities were commonly felt to be the one method which allowed for discovery rather than relied upon passive reporting.[5]

In England street visits formed an important part of the rationale for dividing Unions into medical districts within each of which a designated doctor should build up a detailed knowledge of the condition of the population and of the risks therein to public health. However, gathering such knowledge was painstaking and labour-intensive and was usually more than all but the most dedicated Union medical officers could achieve. In Plymouth and East Stonehouse it was revealing how quickly Kay and McClure became the local experts and how from their scientific curiosity and work with the families of seamen and marines they acquired a clearer map of the districts than any of the city's doctors. Chadwick observed the same weakness in the system in London, where metropolitan policemen were soon identified as by far the most effective sources of information for the Boards of Health. The police force, five thousand strong, was the only organisation which covered the whole city; conversely, Chadwick noted, medics and inspectors of nuisances were 'solitary men dotted here and there'.[6] In any event, there was no legal or official benchmark against which to judge whether a Board of Health or Union Guardians had taken reasonable care to find and treat all those within their boundaries. Undoubtedly some among the sick poor remained undetected even in Plymouth, where Beer and Morrish worked alongside practitioners engaged by the Board of Health. In East Stonehouse, by common consent, the authorities were judged to have fallen well short of expectation.

The General Board of Health did distinguish between cleansing offensive property in the interests of the public at large and treating individuals. It stipulated that Union Guardians should dispense free medicine for the poor while cholera continued which, it was hoped, would cure any mild attack and hence forestall later hospital admission. But effectiveness was limited by the unwillingness or inability of those who suffered both to acknowledge initial symptoms and to come forward to receive help. Convenient dispensing outlets were obviously crucial, as the Navy recognised independently of any steps taken by the civic authorities in the three towns. Rae and Nicolas were convinced that distributing medicine among naval employees in this way was worthwhile and they promptly set up a dispensing post at the gates of the victualling yard. For the Royal Naval Hospital this was a first line of defence against the prospect of uncontrolled numbers suddenly requiring admission, many of whom would be too ill to be saved. Rae was a firm advocate of pre-emptive measures and early treatment whose experience led him to believe that delayed access to medical care was costing many lives. A carminative mixture, prepared at the naval hospital's dispensary, was left with the police and directions given about how it should be taken. This was both an economical and effective plan, Rae calculated; surely nothing could be better than handing out free medicine at a place of work which so many labourers attended? Events indeed appeared to justify his confidence. A later Governor recalled how the health of the men employed at the victualling yard had benefited greatly from Rae's mixture.[7] Successful as Rae may have been, however, his medicine was available only to those who worked at the yard, who were not likely to be among the poorest or destitute of the population.

The problem of reaching all sections of society was explained by Soltau in a public lecture in Plymouth later in the year. As a doctor and leading member of the Plymouth Board of Health, Soltau recollected how after the Union had been divided into fourteen medical districts, each with its practitioner to tend to the poor and with placards everywhere warning of the dangers of ignoring premonitory symptoms of cholera, and indicating where free medicines and advice could be obtained, the lower orders remained oblivious to the peril facing them. The poor, Soltau concluded, could or would not recognise the illness until the victim collapsed and death became the likely outcome. 'This was the history of almost every fatal case which I attended,' he continued. Ignorance and irresponsibility thereby inevitably went far to account for the fate of so many.

Lest such an explanation be thought suspiciously convenient, Soltau delved into the psychology of the poorest classes so as to demonstrate their remoteness from even the best-conceived medical plans. It was not just that they could not be bothered, hoped that any sense of unease would pass or that they attached no importance to any symptoms where pain and cramps were absent. The poor were also superstitious in their distrust of doctors and of the scientific knowledge which professionals brought to bear. 'There existed in the minds of many of the lower orders a firm conviction that the remedies administered in cholera put patients into a sleep from whence they never awoke,' Soltau declared. When prescribing he had frequently been asked 'whether the pill I had given them was one of *those* pills about which there had been so much talk'.[8] To the untrained eye the rapid collapse which marked an advanced case of Asiatic cholera was similar to the stupor induced by opiates; it was also possible that this association led the uninformed to think that it was the remedy rather than the disease itself which produced such striking effects.

Nevertheless, underlying this was an ingrained distrust of those in positions of authority which was shared by all sections of the working class until the later decades of the nineteenth century. In the minds of the poor, middle-class intrusions into their living conditions were just a further means of control. Widespread among the poor was the conviction that the practitioners sent among them were paid by the civic authorities only for cases which proved fatal and therefore that medical officers made their living by killing off as many useless paupers as possible.[9] Chadwick certainly knew that the whole system of medical relief had to operate within a hostile culture. 'The belief has now gone out that the doctors are poisoning the wells,' he despaired in September 1849;[10] many paupers had instinctively regarded the excitement about cholera as an opportunity for Poor Law Guardians to do their worst. Such fears had found expression in violent disturbances, as in Manchester, in 1832 when the new Anatomy Act and an epidemic which killed so many appeared to be too much of a coincidence.

Soltau's remarks indicated that it had not been possible to break down these suspicions in the three towns; that did not mean, though, that considerable progress in tackling fundamental problems in public health had not been made. Soltau described in graphic detail the dirt, bad ventilation and appalling overcrowding which health officials had discovered in Plymouth and he urged his audience to pay greater attention to the way in which the poor lived in the worst districts, since these were the breeding grounds not only for cholera but also for typhus, fevers, smallpox, measles and scarlatina. Judging the past year, he lauded the Plymouth Board of Health for what had been achieved. In its efforts to reach all in need it had even provided round-the-clock help for suspected cholera sufferers at the Guildhall, where throughout each night one medical officer sat up on duty and where on four nights the conscientious Soltau also took his turn responding to emergencies. This was a further pointer to how seriously members of his Board took their obligations.

But for all the much-vaunted provisions made by the authorities, Plymouth's paupers were still largely dependent on charitable work for tangible benefit. Charity was, of course, well established in Britain; the country's poor were certainly more familiar with traditional patterns of patronage than they were with the newer, more formal structures emanating from reforming legislation. Indeed, understanding how the poor were helped in early-Victorian Britain required even more than an acquaintance with the institutions set up by benefactors to which they might apply. Informal systems built via kinship and community could often determine whether recourse to organised assistance was necessary in the first place, let alone the amount required. Help at this level might also come from philanthropic visiting by middle-class women who, moved by religious conviction or social obligation, offered both moral and material support in the home and in a manner which often minimised the stigma which attached to hardship.[11] Such visits, although they might provide elementary advice, food and blankets, seldom brought medical care; for that the poor would have to look elsewhere, at which point the limitations of institutional charities were sometimes soon revealed. When cholera took hold in Plymouth, for instance, the South Devon and East Cornwall Hospital's management committee resolved at once to refuse all cases on the grounds that its very restricted accommodation would be overwhelmed. The authorities in the three towns 'most liberally and energetically provided for the destitute poor who were attacked by the disease', its secretary explained. To take cholera patients would divert this charitable foundation from its legitimate purpose.[12]

Fortunately for those denied succour at the South Devon and East Cornwall Hospital, the emergency public dispensaries, and in particular the Plymouth Public Dispensary, proved far better ports of call. At the latter, Cookworthy not only doled out medicines to cholera victims but with his assistants managed to visit patients in their homes. It was his boast that up to 31 August 1849 only one cholera case treated by the dispensary had died. Valuable as this work was, no dispensary could hope to offer the nursing so essential in cholera cases, nor was it really possible for any Board of Health to do so beyond that available at a designated cholera hospital. In 1832 the Exeter Corporation of the Poor had experimented with visiting nurses by engaging twenty-four of them at 2/6d per diem. That number, however, was never likely to prove sufficient.[13] Cost was invariably a great inhibitor. A few Boards of Guardians in London in 1849 voted money for some nursing in the community but others, as at Tooting where the epidemic was severe and at Bethnal Green where the General Board of Health specifically requested their employment, refused.[14] But money was not the only difficulty. The women who generally were available for such work were usually both untrained and unsuitable: even in hospitals standards were low and turnover high while in workhouse infirmaries nursing tasks perforce devolved to able-bodied paupers. Despite some voluntary initiatives to raise the profile of nursing in the 1840s, recognised training and a professional ethos did not begin to develop until the 1860s and the advent of Florence Nightingale as an icon of the Victorian era.[15]

For those among the poor of the south Devon towns confined to their own miserable dwellings, the only care beyond that of family and neighbours came from the dedicated and much-publicised labours of the Society of Sisters of Mercy of the Holy Trinity. These were women from Lydia Sellon's Anglican foundation of nursing sisters who had joined with her in order to work among the poor in Devonport in 1848. Sellon was the stong-willed, twenty-seven-year old daughter of a naval commander and committed to the re-establishment of vocational religious life in post-Reformation Britain. Her efforts were a visible aspect of early-Victorian, high-church revival and followed from the successful founding of the Park Village Sisters in 1845 and the St John's nursing order in London earlier in 1848.[16] But such vocational orders inevitably attracted suspicion. They were viewed as too close in lifestyle and religious practices to their Roman counterparts and even as subversive instruments for the spread of Catholicism. Although patronised by some high-church clergy and remaining within the Anglican communion, they provoked controversy by sporting prominent badges and obstinacy in the face of secular authority, which made them generally unwelcome as hospital volunteers.[17]

Latimer was certainly vigilant of the Sisters' activities around Plymouth. The *Journal* reported warily on the home for orphans which they ran in Devonport and stressed how vulnerable children were to religious indoctrination.[18] Some children who had left the orphanage had reputedly witnessed the crosses the women wore beneath their dresses and how a statue of the Virgin was venerated within the building. Readers were even urged to be distrustful of clergy who associated with the order, since on doctrinal matters all sympathisers were alarmingly vague or silent. Yet as cholera spread and the devotion of the

Sisters for the sick poor in their homes became apparent, Latimer both reflected and encouraged a change in public sentiment and almost acknowledged his harshness in the past. On 19 July his paper praised the Sisters' excellent work when nursing a stricken family through the night and when, amid the worst abodes of Stonehouse Lane, Sellon had come out to make an assessment of need and returned at once with three assistants to tend sick children in special tents erected nearby.

Further commendations of the Sisters for their heroic work were to follow. Not only did they nurse the ill and dying in the worst districts of the city but, since its construction, they had also provided care at the five-fields hospital, where one of the young women succumbed to cholera.[19] The Sisters collected bedding and clothing for distribution among the needy; they presented women recovering from cholera with fresh clothes and in some instances even refurnished rooms in the slums where the victims lived. From the Royal Naval Hospital, Nicolas appeared to confirm that all the *Journal*'s observations were correct. A staunchly orthodox Anglican, he was none the less unstinting in his tribute to the selfless way in which the Sisters nursed by day and by night throughout the epidemic. 'Nothing', he avowed to Burnett, 'can exceed their zeal and constant attendance on the sick.'[20]

Comment on the work of the Sisters of Mercy increasingly stood out as free from the political acrimony and accusations of self-interest which characterised the often critical accounts of the local authorities. More surprisingly, perhaps, it also stood out in contrast with the highly adverse reports about the behaviour of members of the medical profession. By the autumn of 1849 it was clear that many of the suspicions which the poor harboured against practitioners were not without foundation. Close investigation indeed suggested that for all the legislation of recent years and the show of activity by the Plymouth Board of Health, the town's poor were in fact no better served than when trusting to old-fashioned benevolence.

While it was natural for Soltau to ridicule distrust of his profession as an aspect of underclass culture born essentially of ignorance, as a member of the Board of Health he was also anxious to find a diversion from the public outcry which had arisen in the course of the summer about the way in which medical officers were remunerated and the scandalous relationship between his Board and some of Plymouth's druggists. Payment of both practitioners and druggists was usually a matter for contention with all Union Guardians and ratepayers. This, it transpired, had been a factor in the administrative deadlock in Dumfries in 1848 where, Chadwick noted, the parish authorities were 'in fierce conflict with the medical men on the subject of fees'.[21] Doctors were viewed sceptically as being beneficiaries from the fear and publicity of disease and not from its suppression hidden from the common gaze. Like most others, Plymouth's commercial community was alert to panic-mongering among health officers and irresponsible coverage in the press and took exception to the numerous placards advising people to rush for medicine. Such alarm frightened away visitors on business or traders coming to market. Shopkeepers and merchants began to question the growing varieties of cholera with which medical men sought to bamboozle Guardians and ratepayers in order to augment their own employment. What was the difference between cholera, Asiatic cholera, malignant cholera, choleraic diarrhoea or just familiar bowel and stomach upset? The differences were not necessarily those of clinical diagnoses; rather, it was suspected, they lay in the terms of employment of the district medical officers.

The Guardians of the Plymouth Union, through the Plymouth Board of Health, paid the surgeons of the fourteen medical districts half a guinea for each case of cholera up to a maximum fee of ten guineas per district per week. To claim the maximum remuneration a practitioner therefore required twenty cholera diagnoses weekly. There was no payment for treating diarrhoea such as was common in Plymouth every summer. The temptation to diagnose every humble bowel disorder as a variant of cholera was therefore enormous. 'Let the Plymouth doctors say what they like,' one furious ratepayer wrote to Latimer on 6 August, 'not one out of that body, who have been so active in creating alarm, increasing the local taxation, and paralysing the trade of the town, perhaps, ever saw a case of decided Asiatic cholera.'[22] This had not been the manner of payment during the 1832 epidemic when, not surprisingly, the number of diagnosed cases was only half the 1849 levels. Furthermore, it differed from the way in which the district surgeons in East Stonehouse or Devonport were currently being paid. But it was not only for pecuniary gain that the practitioners working for the Plymouth Board of Health inflated the number of cholera cases; they also generated good publicity, and hence in all probability future patronage, by being able to point to success as measured by their much lower death rates among so-called cholera victims than elsewhere. 'What a puff for all the district parish surgeons,' the press pronounced. 'This is fudge!'[23]

Then there was the matter of double charging at the cholera hospital, which came to light at a meeting of the Guardians on 2 August. Fox and Prance were each paid two guineas per day for their labours at the five-fields site, but they were also district surgeons and hence for many of their patients they were being paid in two separate capacities. No one criticised their dedication; indeed Beer stood up to defend them as men of the highest professional standards who risked their own lives every day in a place where already nine of the nursing staff had died. But critics did point out that so many patients at the hospital were mysteriously always convalescing that they might benefit from a 'cook more than a doctor'.[24] Dubious claims from practitioners did not stop there. Another asserted that in order to attend the forty cholera cases in his district he needed a horse and gig to be provided at the Board of Health's expense. This ruse was exposed by a prosperous resident who was able to inform the Board that no cholera existed in the area mentioned; so surely did he know this to be accurate that he offered to donate five pounds to the offending medical officer for every genuine case discovered. The poor, it turned out, were not as ignorant of human motivation as Soltau cared to suggest. Even if they knew nothing of these abuses within the payment structure, their distrust of self-professed, dedicated professionals would have been reinforced by John Sherwell's performance in his district of the Plympton St Mary Union. Sherwell was a rude and poorly qualified doctor who had habitually neglected his pauper charges since first engaged in the 1830s, yet because he settled for a modest stipend the Guardians ignored all complaints about him. On 15 August 1849, when called to examine two women attacked by cholera, Sherwell 'was in such a state of intoxication as to be unable to attend'. The women died soon after.[25]

How had the financial regulations of the Plymouth Board of Health come about and why could such blatant abuses not be checked? These were embarrassing questions for, among others, the press, which otherwise of course held up the Plymouth Board as a model for its neighbours. Indeed, only in the Plymouth Union were there any allegations of corruption in 1849. A partial answer to these questions lay in the contrasting local government structures between the three towns. In

East Stonehouse and Devonport the Boards of Guardians were the sole bodies legally charged with matters of public health, whereas Plymouth had separate Improvement Commissioners also with statutory responsibilities for which a rate was collected accordingly. In short, East Stonehouse and Devonport seemed to have firmer delineations of accountability. This may have encouraged the parsimonious approach to public health for which East Stonehouse in particular was so widely criticised, but at the same time it did permit tighter control over expenditure by single and confident public bodies. The specific complaint in Plymouth was that, the Guardians being less assured of their legal standing and under constant scrutiny, the Board of Health had fallen into the hands of medical practitioners, chemists and druggists who exploited ambiguities and uncertainties to their own financial advantage.

To manifest their concern for public health and as if to broadcast their legitimate responsibility the Plymouth Guardians accepted unquestioningly whatever medical recommendations were placed before them, thereby endorsing the arguments of those members of the Board of Health who had an obvious self-interest. In practice, the business of the Board soon came to be settled by a conclave of medical men deciding among themselves. This was an outrageous abuse in the opinion of many residents. If the forty-two practitioners of Plymouth had volunteered their services gratis in this time of crisis their credibility as disinterested professionals would undoubtedly have been greater. But in fact, as one irate correspondent to the *Journal* pointed out, only eighteen had offered to attend the poor even under the generous terms of employment extended by the Board of Health. Those engaged in the fourteen medical districts were simply jobbing on the poor rate: with a guaranteed expenditure of 140 guineas every week on their fees 'would cholera ever disappear from Plymouth after this?' This was in contrast to Devonport, it was reported a month later, where the Guardians had formed a proper Board of Health and not a board of doctors. Medical staff there were directed by a Board of Health 'firm in the power they possess by law'. The Devonport Guardians were held up to be 'really men of business' among whom there was 'no fawning to another class of officials'.[26]

Disagreements and jealousies among the practitioners who controlled the Plymouth Board of Health were common knowledge, but it was not until mid-August 1849 that one of them, Edward Roe, broke ranks and eventually exposed the extent of malpractice. Roe was a senior and respected Plymouth doctor with a large private practice beyond his current service for the poor as one of the district surgeons. He was none the less part of the payment racket, reporting 123 cholera cases in his district in the six weeks to the end of August – enough but no more than the number required for the maximum ten-guineas-per-week fee. He stayed silent about the Board's irregularities until on 10 August it adopted a proposal to open a second cholera hospital in Plymouth. Roe took up the cause of 200 nearby householders who naturally objected to a site chosen in a densely populated and bustling area close to the workhouse, and on 13 August he presented their petition to his colleagues at the Board of Health and asked for a special meeting to consider the plan. The Board delayed implementation but when the full complement of medical officers and druggists assembled on 30 August Roe's objections to the proposal were ridiculed and permission to proceed was duly granted.

Professionally slighted, Roe resigned from the Board and wrote to Latimer. He now turned upon the Board of Health as being 'forced by the solicitations of one medical man to do an act which the town has already pronounced as most prejudicial to its commercial interests, as most murderous to the lives of the inhabitants'. The town already had a perfectly good cholera hospital at five fields, he insisted, which cost £60 per week to run, yet the doctors and nurses of which had never been overwhelmed and at the time of writing had only sixteen inmates. Roe also wrote to the General Board of Health in London enclosing all the evidence which would prove his case. 'And what drove the Board to sanction a second hospital?' he enquired rhetorically. 'Because a surgeon apothecary, who merely derives his influence from his being a *member* of the Board, has insisted upon it,' he thundered. 'He saves himself trouble, as he can see 50 patients under one roof as quickly as he can ten scattered in various houses!'[27]

Professional antagonisms also played a part in revealing the benefits which certain druggists and chemists in Plymouth derived from their influence as members of the Board of Health. Once more, the antics of the self-righteous middle classes would have come as no surprise to the poor, who held this class of tradesmen in the same contempt as doctors, both being in collusion to syphon money by any opportunity for jobbery. Pharmacy, like medicine, had expanded in early-nineteenth-century Britain and by the 1840s specialist schools provided courses which gave those qualified the trappings of professional status. Chemists often recommended as well as sold concoctions for specific ailments, giving cheaper and direct access to remedies for a large section of the working class. The Pharmaceutical Society had 2,000 members within a year of its foundation in 1841. There was no record of chemists and druggists in Plymouth in the 1840s, although towns of comparable size indicated probable numbers. Exeter, with a population of only 31,000 had fifty-six druggists and chemists. Nottingham's 53,000 people supported ninety, while the 62,000 inhabitants of Norwich had seventy-seven. Sheffield, with almost twice the latter's population in 1841, fared worse with the same total of fifty-six as for Exeter.[28]

Whenever a local Board of Health was constituted and when Guardians engaged and apportioned practitioners to medical districts within their Union, arrangements had to be made for dispensing the medicines prescribed to the poor at the ratepayers' expense. Scope for corruption always existed but Plymouth became a glaring example whereby the three leading druggists of the town, being members of the Board, simply divided up the profitable districts between them, allowing only a few others to participate in this supply. Other chemists and druggists understandably wanted to know why the business of provision for the poor was not open to all. Not only was the favoured ring taking all the trade associated with cholera but, by obliging the poor to go to them now for their subsidised medicines, established ties and loyalties were being disrupted which might never return. All chemists and druggists in Plymouth paid rates to the public authorities and all should be treated by those authorities in the same way. Morrish questioned the legality of existing arrangements at a special meeting of Guardians on 20 August. Why was one member of the Board of Health presenting a bill for £35 on account of supplying medicine to the poor? 'At all events,' Morrish argued, 'their favours might be a little distributed and not all conferred upon one individual.' But the chairman of the meeting refused to take the item: it was out of his power to intervene, he quickly responded. 'The medical men sent where they liked for their medicines.' He would not attempt to control them.[29]

Such was the outcry, however, that the payment system had to be altered. In any case, it was illegal for Poor Law Guardians to contract for or to sell goods either directly or indirectly while responsible for the expenditure of a public rate and those involved eventually realised the need to protect themselves against prosecution. Nevertheless, given the resentment felt by druggists excluded from the ring, this could not he done without a good deal of hostile publicity. Under the original arrangements for reimbursement the chemists and druggists presented their weekly bills directly to the Plymouth Guardians and then validated their own expenses by ensuring endorsement of them by the Board of Health. Under pressure for better scrutiny, modifications in procedure required that the accounts should be presented via district surgeons who would be able to claim the money as for medicines which they had supplied, remitting the sums later to the druggists by way of discharge of private debt. 'Is this to screen the Guardian druggists from the penalty attached to the abuse of office?' one of Plymouth's smaller chemists demanded to know.[30] No other explanation was either possible or indeed forthcoming. However, the complainant observed, the dodge could not work since six of the fourteen district medical officers were qualified as physicians, not surgeons, and hence under the rules of the Royal College of Physicians they could not supply medicines for which to submit a claim. This dispute rumbled on into the winter of 1849. By then a final fraud had come to light concerning supplies to the five-fields hospital.

'The eyes of all ratepayers are now open to the jobbing of Guardian doctors and Guardian druggists,' a correspondent to the *Journal* affirmed. On top of all that had been exposed during the summer the hospital scandal came as a last and sad reflection on the integrity of the medical profession. The cholera hospital, erected so efficiently and where the Sisters of Mercy had long toiled, had been acclaimed as among the finest achievements during the epidemic in Plymouth; no one had ever questioned that it was well supplied to meet the needs of the sick poor. But it emerged that it had been grossly over-supplied with many quite unnecessary medical provisions. 'Chalk medicine with other ineffectual stuff called medicines were by bucketsful sent up to the hospital,' the *Journal* relayed. Ratepayers also wanted to know the whereabouts of a great deal of surplus material which had gone missing when it should have been returned to the Guardians for open auction. All the things removed from five fields were public property, one ratepayer pointed out, yet 'notwithstanding the doctors are to be so well paid, have been taken possession of by a certain doctor to fit up or to add to his surgery'. The Plymouth Guardians were once more condemned for the lack of control which the Board of Health had exercised over grasping medical officers and suppliers. 'They are too *pliant* and submitted to the dictation of the medical men,' the same correspondent charged.[31] If ever Plymouth should be afflicted with cholera again it was to be hoped that the Guardians would treat that profession with more firmness and discernment.

To the dismay of Plymouth's citizens, having shown signs of abating at the end of August and in the fortnight which followed, cholera flared up again after 14 September. East Stonehouse and Devonport were more fortunate. The worst-affected areas this time proved to be in Benbow's district either side of Exeter Street, where old and overcrowded houses had always made their occupants vulnerable. It was indeed remarkable that this district had not suffered more during the heat of July and August when attention had been focused on the other side of the city around Stonehouse Lane. Such drains as the Improvement Commissioners had constructed in the vicinity of Exeter Street emptied into nearby Sutton Pool which, like the Yealm estuary at Noss, became transformed at low tide into a shallow of night soil and decaying waste.

Cases of cholera and choleraic diarrhoea in Plymouth suddenly rose from twenty-six and twenty-nine on 13 and 14 September respectively to sixty-seven on 16 September and 106 on 17 September. Deaths had correspondingly risen from five and two on 13 and 14 September respectively to eighteen on 16 September and twenty-nine on 18 September. Faced with an unexpected emergency, the Board of Guardians appropriated a building for use as a house of refuge and then quickly converted it into a second cholera hospital. Once the outbreak seemed to be contained patients were transferred to the five-fields site, but this was not before near panic had erupted at the Board of Health. Soltau later recalled how within a twenty-four-hour period up to forty cases had been diagnosed around Exeter Street and how amid the chaos he had attended victims there on 15 September. Yet even before that date there had, in fact, been little reliable statistical evidence to suggest that cholera was really disappearing despite the optimistic tone of the press. In the preceding week over 300 new cases had been identified in Plymouth and sixty-three cholera deaths recorded. In Devonport 117 deaths were ascribed to the epidemic during the week to 13 September. East Stonehouse reported nine cholera fatalities in the same period. After 14 September the figures just became worse. Eighty-seven victims died during the week ending 18 September – Plymouth's highest total for any week throughout the 1849 epidemic. In the following seven days sixty more died from among 195 fresh cases.

Whether or not Soltau was correct in attributing the resurgence of disease in Plymouth in mid-September to the living conditions of those most affected, his observations certainly could not explain a simultaneous and dramatic wave of cholera to the west in Cornwall. The epidemic had not spread along the south coast of Cornwall until late in July 1849, but when it finally arrived, as at Mevagissey, its effects were as devastating as anywhere in Britain. The River Tamar separated Devonport from the St Germans Union, which was a sprawling collection of fourteen parishes, presided over by twenty-four elected Poor Law Guardians, containing the towns of Saltash in the north and Torpoint to the east, where the Union's workhouse was located. When conducting his inspections, Gulson, predictably, had found fault with various aspects of the Guardians' management but overall it was a reasonably well-regulated Union which had provided relief, both indoor and outdoor, for well over a thousand paupers, women and children included, annually since the early 1840s. Unlike many of their counterparts across the country the St Germans Guardians had resigned themselves to the inevitability of a cholera epidemic from an early date and in the autumn of 1848 formed a committee to supervise nuisance removals, began circulating to its parish medical officers all notices received from the General Board of Health, and put up posters to warn the community generally of the need for vigilance and cleanliness. Early in 1849 the Union was divided into five medical districts with a parish surgeon appointed for each. As soon as cholera was identified on 20 July at least one public dispensary was set up in all fourteen parishes and suitable spots were examined for both a cholera hospital and a house of refuge.[32] The Guardians of St Germans certainly had persuasive arguments when claiming that there was nothing more they could have done by way of preparation and response to the arrival of the disease.

Nevertheless, by mid-August the Torpoint workhouse had suffered ten deaths from cholera with a further three in the surrounding town, while in Saltash the epidemic had claimed seven more lives. Dr C. W. Chubb, the surgeon in charge of the Torpoint medical district, was himself too ill to tend the sick and no cover could be found from Devonport or Plymouth, where all practitioners were already overworked. Torpoint and its workhouse struggled by with the help of an old naval surgeon who had retired locally and supervisory visits from a physician who lived in Devonport. They eradicated the illness from the workhouse and kept the cholera hospital in operation and when Chubb returned to duty in the last week of August there was a general sense, reported by the Guardians to the Poor Law Board in London, that the epidemic had been successfully extinguished. As in Plymouth, however, the lull was short-lived. On 1 September Chubb reported thirty-one new cases and twelve recent deaths; almost every house in Torpoint was now affected by either full-blown cholera or severe diarrhoea.

No longer able to cope, the Guardians of St Germans turned to the Royal Navy for assistance. They had, in fact, approached the Port Admiral three weeks earlier and been told that in the event of a collapse of medical provision across the Tamar estuary a naval medical officer might be detached from duty for temporary cover and, this being now the case, they wrote to the Royal Naval Hospital. Nicolas responded promptly by sending his two cholera experts, Bowden and McClure, who at once set about cleansing Torpoint and treating the afflicted. Bowden was recalled within a week due to rising admissions at the naval hospital, but McClure stayed on to advise the St Germans Board of Health and, most valuably, to organise the same house-to-house visitations to check both for sick inhabitants and for health nuisances as he had undertaken so successfully in Plymouth and East Stonehouse in the first two weeks of August. Regarding the efforts of Bowden and McClure, 'the Guardians have done everything that has been suggested', the *Journal* observed on 6 September, and the two men were credited with having suppressed the new outbreak.[33] Nicolas also supplied Torpoint with fresh water from the naval victualling yard since local supplies had become inadequate. Meanwhile McClure carried on removing health nuisances from the streets, whitewashing houses and applying copious quantities of Burnett's chloride of zinc in the dwellings of the poorest inhabitants.

Torpoint, however, was not the only settlement on the Cornish coast overwhelmed by the epidemic and for which help from the Navy was desperately needed. To the south were two fishing villages, Kingsand and Cawsand, which in the last days of August had been stunned by twenty-two sudden cholera fatalities. These villages were in the third medical district of the St Germans Union, but within a few days of the outbreak were left with no care when the resident doctor collapsed and subsequently died from the disease. Responding to the pleas of the Guardians, Nicolas sent two assistant-surgeons attached to the naval hospital, Gruggen and William Hambly, to take charge of the epidemic there while a third, Preston, was despatched to help elsewhere in the Union. By 6 September Kingsand, which bore the brunt of the outbreak, had lost sixty inhabitants out of a total population of no more than 600. The final death toll from these two small villages was 111. Not surprisingly, the Guardians were profuse in their gratitude to Nicolas and wrote in glowing terms of the zealous and efficient work of all the young men sent to tend the sick and to check the spread of disease. Silver snuff boxes were presented by local Boards of Health to four of the assistant-surgeons from the naval hospital who worked in different coastal villages and Nicolas commended Bowden and McClure in particular to the Board of Admiralty. At Noss and Torpoint Bowden and McClure had been volunteers from the first, Nicolas explained, and they had shown no reservations about assignments which placed their own lives in danger. Burnett, of course, was quick to draw this exemplary work of naval medical staff to the attention of the Lords of the Admiralty, who could not in any event fail to appreciate the excellent publicity which the Royal Naval Hospital's efforts had generated.

After its peak in the third week of September 1849 cholera subsided rapidly both in the south Devon towns and across the Tamar. At the start of October the Plymouth Board of Health still recorded 143 new victims with twenty-five fatalities, while the Devonport and East Stonehouse authorities reported twenty-four and seven deaths respectively, but the daily drop in cases was so marked that after 4 October there was felt to be no need to publish further statistics. Many of the arrangements made by the local Boards of Health were by this time being quickly dismantled. Some, in fact, had gone even earlier. So successfully had cholera been eradicated at Noss that the Plympton St Mary Guardians had dispensed with Spencer's services and settled his bill for £78 at the beginning of August and then discharged a junior practitioner who had been helping out with a cheque for sixty-nine guineas a week later. A few days afterwards *Ringdove* was recalled from the Yealm estuary and the Guardians were ordered to arrange for the ship's thorough cleansing before collection.[34] Like Plympton St Mary, the Stoke Damerel Union largely escaped the return of cholera in September and in Devonport the Board of Health resolved to reduce its medical staff on 18 September.

The Plymouth Board of Health could take no such step until a week into October, when it too announced that the contracts with its fourteen district medical officers would be terminated and that any remaining cholera cases would be dealt with at parish level or in the workhouse in the normal way. No sailor or marine was diagnosed with cholera after that time and the last cholera admission to the Royal Naval Hospital took place on 26 September. By 25 October all the additional naval surgeons and assistants sent both there and to the Royal Marine Infirmary had been returned to half pay. Only a handful of measures were retained. The Guardians of Plympton St Mary continued to hold weekly meetings until April 1850 before reverting to the fortnightly norm, while in Devonport, once the Board of Health ceased to function, the Borough's Watch Committee agreed to send policemen to help with occasional house visitations.[35] But these were merely tokens. By the middle of October it was obvious to everyone in Plymouth, Devonport, East Stonehouse and the surrounding villages that the epidemic was over. The recriminations, by contrast, would continue for months to come.

CHAPTER 10

Conclusion

When the official statistics were compiled in the winter of 1849 Plymouth was adjudged to have lost 819 citizens to cholera from among the 3,360 cases diagnosed. With fatalities from Devonport and East Stonehouse included, the total for the naval towns came to 1,894. Cholera deaths in the adjacent Unions of Plympton St Mary and St Germans, when added, took the aggregate for the area in a ten-mile radius of Plymouth to 2,381.[1] Within just three months the region had sustained about 4 per cent of Britain's cholera deaths during the whole of the 1848–49 epidemic. Gulson was aware that his district suffered more intensely than most. When approving final payments to the extra medical officers engaged by the Plympton St Mary Guardians in November 1849 he reminded the Poor Law Board that 'cholera was more severe in the district referred to than in any other part of England of which I have seen any account'.[2]

In contrast to the epidemic of 1832, which officially claimed the lives of 1,031 persons across the three towns, that of 1849 was not restricted to the slums. The chairman of the Devonport Improvement Commissioners and the surveyor of the Plymouth Town Council both succumbed to the disease in 1849; so clearly had cholera broken out this time beyond the courts and alleys where the poor resided that up to 5,000 of Plymouth's more respectable inhabitants may have fled the city. Those who had struggled against the scourge felt an enhanced spirit of community which seemed to transcend social divisions and to supersede the fractiousness of municipal politics. Relief funds had been set up, collections made in well-attended churches and committees constituted for the purpose of visiting and distributing clothing to the afflicted poor. Prominent families subscribed generously to these charitable projects, the *Journal* assured its readers. In the Stoke Damerel Union, which recorded 779 fatalities from 2,155 cholera cases, the chairman of the Board of Health likewise reflected stoically that 'something above a mercenary spirit has prevailed'.[3]

This rhetoric of conciliation found political expression when in November 1849 the Liberal majority on the Plymouth Town Council offered the annual mayoralty to a senior Tory Councillor who had worked publicly on behalf of cholera victims in recent months. The offer was declined, as Liberals may have known it would be, but even Latimer supported this gesture towards healing rifts in the city's politics. There had been no Tory mayor since 1832 and to that extent the Liberals had indeed offered a high-profile political rehabilitation to their long-discredited opponents. More prosaically, the Council reviewed its public health provisions in the wake of the epidemic and for a time a greater sense of urgency was apparent. A special committee to review street cleaning and the removal of night soil from the city was set up in December 1849, the Water Committee endorsed cutting a culvert to improve the flow and the dispersal of nuisances from one of the city's principal waste leats, while Plymouth's Improvement Commissioners recommended purchasing premises where street redevelopment would alleviate congestion. Straightening and widening the streets would naturally be costly, yet the public benefit would be enormous. Old buildings could be demolished which had been 'for many years occupied by prostitutes and disorderly persons wherein cholera lately prevailed to a fearful extent'.[4] Between July and October 1849 the Commissioners met frequently to consider a rising number of requests for drainage inspections and extensions and for the removal of cesspools and dung pits. Most of these were not agreed but tenders were invited for the construction of a new drain at the western end of Stonehouse Lane before it ran into the parish of East Stonehouse.[5]

Drains and roads being predominantly the Commissioners' domain, their surveyor was asked to make an urgent report once the epidemic had subsided. 'The Macadamised roads are extremely dilapidated and filthy,' the Commissioners were starkly informed, 'nor will they be improved until a material of *harder* description is used in repairs.'[6] Where the main streets had been maintained in the past a cheap limestone had been used, the surface of which was prone to turn to mud in winter and to give off clouds of dust in spells of dry weather. Quality stone, though more costly, was the answer, the surveyor urged, and in the long run the bills would be reduced by less frequent repair. As for drains, £3,000 should be spent to build a new main sewer in central Plymouth and a further £2,000 in order to provide sewers of sufficient size for the twenty-seven streets in the town where still no facility existed. Five thousand pounds was a hefty sum to raise yet the surveyor's report was approved and adopted. With so many lives lost due to their perceived negligence over many years there was little else that the Improvement Commissioners could do.

Soul searching also took place in Devonport, where the Board of Health concluded that there was insufficient drainage in the town and that until this was rectified the danger of another epidemic would be ever present. 'Let the cry be Sewerage! Sewerage! Sewerage! till the proper parties attend thereto,' the Board implored, while pleading also for its own existence now that the emergency was over. With its house-to-house inspections, medical officers and nuisance removals the Board had proved its worth; it behoved both the Borough of Devonport and Stoke Damerel authorities now 'to prepare for the future such machinery as may at once be set to work in case of need; whether of cholera, or any other epidemic, endemic, contagious, or infectious disease'.[7] Part of that machinery should be a paid secretary, whose job it would be to organise the enforcement of cleanliness across the Union. Another essential for the increased population of Devonport was a larger supply of pure water. Beyond that, the Board urged the Borough Council to address the overcrowded and overbuilt state of several parts of Devonport where the worst properties should be bought up and then razed to the ground with stringent clauses inserted in any new leases to prevent the recurrence of such abuses. This would carry the work of local government into largely uncharted territory and was not perhaps a realistic exhortation. But in the winter of 1849 the shock of recent months had left a climate of opinion in which almost anything which might avert another calamity was at least given a hearing.

It was not long, though, before reflection turned to recrimination. Vested interest coloured most accounts of what had led to so severe an epidemic and why those charged with safeguarding public health had been so unprepared: those most outspoken were usually anxious to shift the focus of attention as far from their own responsibilities as possible. In Plymouth Soltau had to exonerate himself and his professional colleagues on the Board of Health and to sidestep the widespread criticism of corruption. In Devonport the Board of Health likewise needed to justify its performance during the summer of 1849. The Board 'sustained a very onerous burden on behalf of their fellow parishioners', its chairman declared. With the benefit of hindsight some things might have been done differently, he acknowledged, 'but actions, not words, were needful and they feel they have done the best the circumstances of the case permitted'.[8] These circumstances he was eager to define: they were not the lifestyles of the poor, such as the Plymouth Board emphasised, but rather the habits of a class of men easily identifiable but without many friends on to whose shoulders blame could plausibly be pushed: landlords.

Having already criticised the want of adequate sewerage in the Borough, the Devonport Board of Health now adroitly pointed out that many holders of property seemed entirely oblivious to their social duties. The greed of landlords produced multi-occupancy slums which in turn became the breeding grounds for disease. The press was also quick to turn on those who made a living by letting scanty accommodation to the poor. Such men cared nothing for the lives of others; their only concern was to cram in as many tenants as any house could hold. With the epidemic over, Latimer warned with menace: 'these mercenary landlords have to answer for their shortcomings'. If cholera had brought one benefit, 'it has shown us how hardly the poor are trampled upon – how little they are cared for'.[9] This was good radical rhetoric, but it did not touch upon the real issue of housing stock, which most agreed was in urgent need of improvement and which had conspicuously failed to increase in line with rapid population expansion during the past half century.

Yet the lifestyles of the poor and the avarice of landlords aside, it was the institutions of local government which bore the brunt of public anger. Improvement Commissioners were held accountable for the decaying state of the urban infrastructure, at least in Plymouth and Devonport where Local Acts applied, while the Boards of Guardians had failed to prepare for and to respond to the cholera which by the summer of 1849 had already swept across most of the country. Forming Boards of Health, dividing Unions into medical districts, appointing district medical officers, warning the citizenry of an epidemic, ensuring the removal of nuisances, organising house inspections, erecting cholera hospitals, creating houses of refuge, issuing medicines freely to the poor at public dispensaries and removing the dead from public places were all the responsibilities of Union Guardians. Some Unions, however, were perceived to have undertaken their duties more assiduously than others and throughout the epidemic criticism of the Plymouth and Stoke Damerel Guardians never reached the level reserved for those of East Stonehouse. Cumbersome as the East Stonehouse Guardians may have been, though, the abuse they received was not always justified and Gulson, as an outside observer, saw no yawning gap between the performances of the three authorities. Plymouth doubtless escaped criticism from some quarters, in particular from Latimer, because it had a Liberal-dominated Town Council which, although possessing little legal role, did contribute members to the Board of Health and appeared a beacon of representative democracy under the 1835 Act. Shortcomings in local government, for political reasons, were therefore always more conveniently identified elsewhere.

For advocates of reform the opportunity to attack the Improvement Commissioners as inefficient relics of a bygone age was a godsend. The scope for exploiting antagonism between old and new structures, however, was initially minimised by the fact that many leading figures in the city's public life were members of both and were often happy to smooth over disputes of jurisdiction. But hostility did explode late in the summer of 1849 with a bitterness ill-suited to the conciliatory face which both Liberals and Tories had seemed eager to demonstrate to an anxious population. In August, when the appointment of a new surveyor became a matter of urgency, the clerks of the Improvement Commission and Town Council consulted about whether a joint appointment might be made. At a stormy meeting of the Commissioners the idea was vigorously opposed by those who saw it as the thin end of a wedge being driven into the Commission's historic role by an increasingly assertive municipal authority. 'What was the use of the Commissioners meeting at all if they were bound to choose the man whom the Town Council elected?', one disgruntled officer enquired. 'This was just shoving a person down their throats whether they were willing or not.' But in the end calmer spirits prevailed. The Commission's chairman, Herbert Gibson, had also been elected to the Town Council in 1835 and he and other Commissioners who were Council members could give much-needed reassurance that nothing coercive was intended. The two bodies, whatever their political differences and legal status, the assembly was reminded, 'were like a man and his wife living in the same house'. For the sake of their town it was not good that they should quarrel.[10]

Their quarrels continued none the less. At a Town Council meeting on 19 September the Improvement Commissioners were attacked for their apathy in cleaning and draining the town. Members of the Commission present took strong objection and amid the uproar which ensued the mayor was eventually obliged to rule that he would hear no more discussion along those lines. Gibson later complained of an underhand campaign by political reformers against the Commissioners. When pressed by Council officials the Improvement Commissioners were able to reel off lists of drains built, streets connected and further works either planned or already under way. But the accusations of too little too late and at too great a cost always returned, and not only in Plymouth. The Devonport Board of Health was scathing about the Borough's Improvement Commissioners when it observed that 'large sums of money have been taken from the holders of property for sewers', yet they could discern 'no corresponding results'.[11] As in Plymouth, cholera had exposed the fragmentary nature of local government and conflicts between its institutions.

Beyond highlighting conflicting interests, the epidemic revealed the hopelessly confused structure of local government finances. The costs of cholera fell predominantly on the Boards of Union Guardians, whose capacity to raise money was frequently bounded by the provisions of Local Acts and legal restraints regardless of the more mundane consideration of what might be collectable from reluctant payers of the Poor Rate. The Plymouth Guardians cited £5,000 as the expense additionally incurred in 1849.[12] Since no extra rate could be set nor the recovery of past expenditure imposed upon the ratepayers of future years, borrowing was their only recourse and in September £2,000 was borrowed from a bank. But as Gulson later confirmed: 'it is clearly illegal to borrow money for the purpose of paying the current expenses for the relief of the poor'.[13] The loan and interest due upon it could not therefore be allowed by the district auditor, which in itself prised open old arguments within the Board of Guardians about how money should be raised and spent.

The most forceful critic of financial management was William Mortimer, who had been chairman of the Plymouth Guardians between 1842 and 1846. He was also a prominent Improvement Commissioner and had been elected to the Town Council in 1835. During his tenure the legal loophole of setting successive rates, each to cover only a few months during any one rating year, had been devised and had his clever system been retained after 1847 the financial embarrassment of 1849 might have been avoided. Fundamentally, the legal authority to raise money dated from an age when the sums required were considerably lower; by the late 1840s it was only by exploiting technicalities in the wording of Local Acts that solvency could be maintained. This was no basis for local authority finances, Mortimer complained; the only solution was for the Poor Law Board in London to issue an order for financial restructuring as, he believed, it had the power to do under the 1834 Act. 'Without such, irregularities will prevail,' he warned, '– no uniform practice abided by.'[14]

But did the Poor Law Board really have such powers? The Board itself did not know and when formally confronted with the whole problem of the illegal loan of 1849 and the circumstances which had necessitated it simply responded that it had no authority to interfere. This was effrontery, Harris, as current chairman of the Guardians, explained months later. Much of the expenditure incurred which had made the £2,000 loan so urgent had been at the behest of Milroy, who had been sent down from the General Board of Health specifically to advise the local authorities. It was typical of central government that having stipulated what should be done, when the issue of paying the bills arose it disclaimed all competence. But the chaos over finance extended even beyond these disputes about the rate which could be raised and whether borrowing was legal. Among the Guardians there was no agreed record of what use the £2,000 loan was to be put to. When they met on 29 November Morrish claimed that it was for paying the bills which arose from the emergency measures to combat the epidemic. Not everyone agreed.

Boards of Guardians would commonly deal with problems of cash flow in times of crisis and Plymouth was not unusual in this respect. In Stoke Damerel the cost of the epidemic was put at 'one shilling in the pound on the rated value of the parish', but in the meantime debts had to be settled at once 'as it is not fair on tradesmen of the town to be kept without payment when they are already suffering from a depression of business'.[15] That was also Morrish's argument in Plymouth but Gibson, a Guardian in addition to his other positions of influence, denied that traders had any prior claims. It fell to David Derry, another stalwart member of the Board of Guardians, Improvement Commissioner, Town Councillor since 1835 and chairman of the Council's Finance Committee since 1846, to resolve the disagreement to the evident satisfaction of all. It was calculated that more than £2,000 was owed to the medical practitioners and chemists who had so swayed the Plymouth Board of Health. 'As the druggists and surgeons had done their work at a very large compensation,' he suggested, 'they would not complain if they had to wait a few months for their claims to be met.'[16] It was, needless to say, no solution to the financial crisis but the meeting adjourned with a general sense that no injustice had been done. Derry was elected mayor of Plymouth in 1850.

All these clashes and recriminations not only divided the organs of local government in Plymouth and its neighbouring towns but were also played out in large measure on a public stage. Whatever sense of community and shared danger cholera might have encouraged, legal hearings, special enquiries, open lectures and the constant judgements of the press also kept the fractiousness of local affairs alive and informed the population about the energy displayed by different authorities, the effectiveness of measures taken to contain the epidemic and the ability of those authorities to provide for the sick and the poor as the law required. Latimer set about his task with predictable self-righteousness; his *Journal* became a self-acclaimed voice for the inhabitants of the three towns, exposing vested interest, malpractice and sheer incompetence. Its staff attended and reported meetings and its columns carried letters and editorials scathing in tone. The sufferings of cholera victims and the conditions among which the sick poor lived were graphically recalled, as were heart-rending accounts of individuals moved by concern for their fellow beings to care for others heedless of their own safety – thereby making good the glaring shortcomings in provision by Guardians and Boards of Health. Extolling the innate goodness which might be found among ordinary people, however, was not a ploy reserved just for those who wished to draw a contrast with the performance of responsible bodies.

Soltau also eulogised on what had been done by way of individual sacrifice during the epidemic, but his descriptions conveyed a more subtle message. When he spoke of uplifting examples of humanity it was always via personal observation, thereby illustrating how he, like other officers of the Plymouth Board of Health, had moved constantly among the most afflicted. In fairness to Soltau and the Plymouth authorities, most observers did grant them some successes. The five-fields hospital admitted 228 serious cases between 27 July and 11 September but lost only ninety patients, which spoke well for its medical staff and facilities. Similarly, house-to-house visits in the poorest districts were credited with an improvement in cleanliness and the discovery of many sick in need of treatment. But posturing being an integral part of politics, Soltau knew as well as anyone the advantages of favourable presentation. Concern for the sick and needy featured prominently in his and in the rhetoric of all bodies under pressure to demonstrate that they had done everything possible to fulfil their public health obligations prior to the arrival of the epidemic or everything that could reasonably have been expected once the outbreak was confirmed. As the weeks passed during the summer of 1849 the press had grown in importance as a mouthpiece for, and even at times arbiter between, the competing accusations made by and against Guardians, Commissioners, Boards of Health and medical officers.

Latimer, naturally, was quick to publish letters from all correspondents who were grateful for the *Journal*'s role in exposing negligence and fraud, although his own politics ensured that he was more eager to expose those failings in some quarters than in others. In Plymouth his criticism was largely limited to Improvement Commissioners, whereas in East Stonehouse, traditionally Tory and untouched by the municipal reforms of 1835, no restraints applied. Although there were good grounds for accusing the latter's Board of Health of being ponderous and insensitive, when statistics were considered the incidence of death and disease in East Stonehouse was no worse than in Plymouth and Devonport – yet this point was consistently ignored in all the *Journal*'s coverage. Latimer also consistently belittled the difficulties faced by the East Stonehouse authorities while praising what was done elsewhere against fewer impediments.

Confronted by so doughty a champion of local government reform, the authorities reacted differently to the prospect of newspaper publicity from the outset and sometimes in ways which merely compounded their problems. As Beer and Morrish demonstrated in the

Plymouth Union, a skilful handling of the press paid handsome dividends. Courting its journalist and taking him out into the slums to see public health officials at work was a masterstroke which the Guardians in other Unions would have done well to emulate. Writing of the Plymouth authorities in September 1849 the *Journal* concluded enthusiastically, though with questionable justification, that 'we are glad to state that the Board of Health have been as active and zealous as ever in their endeavours to subdue the plague'. The Board's counterpart in Devonport did manage to improve its press relations somewhat in the course of the summer and eventually earned the modest epithet 'industrious'.[17] But the East Stonehouse authorities never raised their standing. Even with their nuisance removal record gradually improving, they still seemed secretive in the conduct of business and were hopelessly slow in the production of statistical data. Public health matters in East Stonehouse were also overshadowed by the extensive coverage given to the disastrous proceedings relating to dung wharf. A belief that whatever they did would be distorted or ridiculed by a hostile press made the Guardians of East Stonehouse awkward and defensive during litigation or on public occasions. In Plympton St Mary this reticence was even more extreme. There the Guardians refused to allow journalists to attend their meetings, so distrustful were they of the prying eye of popular scrutiny. Among the many challenges which cholera posed for local authorities in the late 1840s was that of the growing importance of openness and press management in an age when public perceptions could be quickly formed. An intrusive press, as became apparent, soon made heroes and villains in any crisis.

Of course, when exposing inactivity and muddle on the part of statutory authorities in south Devon the *Journal* was doing little more than joining the wider criticism of how such bodies functioned the length and breadth of the land. Lord Ashley, looking back on the cholera years, considered that all Boards of Guardians revealed 'their selfishness, their cruelty, their reluctance to meet and to relieve the suffering poor in the days of the epidemic'.[18] Chadwick likewise had no illusions about how even bodies created by the parliamentary legislation which he had inspired had reacted in the crisis. Reflecting on public health and other advances on behalf of the poor in Britain in 1851, he cited not local Boards of Health but the clergy of the Church of England as among the most active and effective proponents. Devon was typical. Most of the county's clergy acted as agents for the Savings Bank at Exeter, they were the trustees and promoters of clothing clubs and they raised the subscriptions necessary for founding and maintaining elementary schools. 'They were the first to take up the cause of sanitary improvement,' Chadwick suggested, 'and are now its best supporters throughout the country,'[19] Given that most Boards of Health were little more than Guardians or Commissioners acting in a different name and were disbanded once the epidemic had passed, it was not perhaps surprising that even Chadwick saw the efforts of committed clergy as a focus for continuity.

It was indeed common to see Union Guardians across the country slipping back into old ways by the autumn of 1849 and the Devon naval towns were no exceptions. From Plymouth, Morrish wrote to the General Board of Health in January 1850 complaining that public health nuisances were no longer being removed as they had been while cholera raged.[20] In East Stonehouse, economy was also the order of the day in 1850 as the newly elected Guardians cut back the poor rate following the heavier demands on the ratepayers of previous years. Plympton St Mary was no different: incredibly, there seemed to be a collapse of all enthusiasm for preventive public health measures at Noss within just five weeks of the last cholera case being diagnosed there. As medical officer, Spencer had gone about the village warning that unless the houses and streets were kept clean the disease might well return, but his admonishments appeared to make no impact. The Plympton Guardians were at work to reduce their Union's medical bills which, they judged, had become excessive during the epidemic. In doing so they displayed a pettiness which almost beggared belief.

As early as August 1849 the Plympton Guardians had cavilled over the cost of emergency assistance for one of its medical officers. Two men had been temporarily engaged to help Dr David Jones with cholera in the Plymstock district but when the Guardians learnt of Jones's extravagance they ruled at once that it must be 'subject to such payment as if only one worked'.[21] They next set about reducing by 10 per cent the remuneration of all Union officials responsible for the care of the poor, which was prevented only when Gulson persuaded the Poor Law Board to intervene in February 1850. Undeterred, the Guardians then turned on their seven district surgeons, allowing a 10 per cent increase in their stipends but on the harsh condition that all claims for the extra work and expenses associated with their duties, such as midwifery calls, were abolished. In practice this would reduce the money paid by 19 per cent and, predictably, no practitioner was prepared to tender for the work on those terms. In the end the old arrangements had to be restored, but again not before the matter had been referred to London. Hopes that the lessons of 1848–49 had been learned, in particular that an annual outlay for prevention was in the long run a smaller expense than the large, sporadic costs of recurring epidemics, seemed to have been dashed in all the south Devon Unions. Within four years the Governor of the Royal Naval Hospital was once more complaining about the foul odours arising from the discharge of sewage and manufacturing waste into the creek close by. In 1853, as in 1849, the Admiralty's lawyers were instructed to serve notice to the Board of Guardians of East Stonehouse for the removal of public health nuisances.

Was it surprising that nothing seemed to have changed? The same structures of authority, the same overlapping responsibilities and the same clashes of interest were still in place when the epidemic died away and the practical problems of effecting change, even where the will existed, soon surfaced again. At first glance, cholera did little to diminish the suspicions of central government interference in local affairs even among men who now conceded that public health provision in the past had been inadequate. The Board of Health in Devonport, reporting on its efforts to the Borough Council towards the end of 1849, summed up this attitude precisely: maintaining itself in being and with a paid secretary in future was justifiable for the very reason that it could effect improvement in the Borough 'without calling in any foreign aid whatever'.[22] The Guardians of the Plymouth Union, quarrelsome and mired as they were in debt following their unscheduled expenditures, almost uniformly resented the opinion handed down from London that the £2,000 borrowed in order to cover day-to-day disbursements had been illegal. They were emphatic in the view that 'they had a right to borrow £2,000 or even £20,000, and that the Poor Law Board had nothing whatever to do with it'.[23] In 1850 they rebutted interference by the General Board of Health in the town's affairs. When meeting as the Board of Health and receiving from London notice that new public health hazards had been reported in places around the town, the Guardians replied that since Plymouth had Improvement Commissioners who held statutory powers in such matters the General Board would do better to write to them since it most certainly had no authority to force the local Board of Health to take any action. It was an inspiring defence of Plymouth's autonomy. Unfortunately it did not address the matter which had led the General Board to write.

The problem of filth piling up again in the town in fact grew worse as the months passed. At the end of 1851 the Plymouth Town Council became involved when a special committee was set up to try to find a solution. The fact that none could be devised demonstrated the practical difficulties which so often frustrated the best efforts of officials. In 1849 two private contractors had been engaged at a cost of £500 per annum to remove the town's night soil and to cleanse the public thoroughfares. The contracts expired in 1852 and given how unsatisfactory the contractors had proved to be it was widely felt that they should not be renewed. But despite repeated public advertisements no one else had tendered. The previous method of removing night soil had been by the Corporation employing pauper labourers and then selling the accumulated waste as agricultural fertiliser. On investigation, however, the market for this had much declined since the mid-1840s and the Council therefore was left with no alternative but to reopen negotiations with those individuals who had performed so poorly in the past.[24] However the local authority might be formed, there were always economic forces at work which played as large a role as any political will in determining its actions.

Beyond the ever present forces of economic reality, local government in Britain after 1849 also remained subjected to a fundamental contradiction affecting the discharge of responsibilities which was quite distinct from the problems of fragmentation and overlapping jurisdictions. This contradiction was most obvious in the differing duties of Boards of Guardians. Charged with operation of the 1834 Poor Law, Guardians were at the same time the instruments of relief for paupers while the collectors of poor rates from those who defined effectiveness by the least possible cost. By forming themselves into Boards of Health in 1848–49 Guardians merely extended the contradiction since accountability to a ratepaying electorate now had also to be balanced against obligations laid down by the legislation of 1848 and the supervisory directions of the General Board of Health. As local Boards of Health, Guardians hoped to keep control over expenditure. This did not work in Plymouth but so well did it succeed in East Stonehouse that Latimer drew residents' attention to what, he argued, was an abuse of power. In order to minimise expenditure the East Stonehouse Board of Health judged flagrant nuisances to public health not to be so; as Guardians, they then did not need to take further action. 'This is not right, or fair or just,' the *Journal* concluded. 'The Board of Guardians were not elected merely to put the screw upon public expenditure but, having constituted themselves into a Board of Health, they were bound to do what they professed it to be their intention to do.'[25]

Guardians too zealous in their help for the poor or who took their duties as members of Boards of Health too seriously invariably risked the wrath of ratepayers. The Guardians of East Stonehouse may have been remiss in preparing the parish for the arrival of cholera as far as Gulson, Nicolas and Latimer were concerned, but even the modest steps taken proved to be unpalatable to the voters. In 1849 Gulson noted how the elections of Guardians had become dominated by short-term parsimony and how any sense of continuity or consensus as to duties seemed to be lost. 'As one party gets in and turns the other out, so the officers are confided in, or otherwise,' he noted disapprovingly. 'All the old Guardians were turned out and a new set elected, pledged to a reduction of expenditure.'[26] Nor did there appear to be any way to circumvent this general problem. When, in 1849, Clitheroe Town Council became so disgusted with its Board of Guardians that it sought for itself powers to charge costs to the town rate, it was informed that it had no legal authority to do so. The General Board of Health ruled that in matters of poor relief and public health 'the Nuisances Act gave the power of charging the rates to the Guardians exclusively'.[27] To the dismay of many reformers, powers of obstruction were even enshrined in their own legislation.

Legal devices, indeed, were often restraints on local initiative. The 1846 and 1848 Nuisances Acts, the 1848 Health of Towns Act and the Public Health Act of 1848 were impressive but, in essence, the legal framework within which Guardians, Health Board officials and government inspectors operated was much the same. To empower the creation of public bodies was not to empower the bodies created, and the limitations of the legislation of the late 1840s were soon apparent even for Chadwick to see: 'I am annoyed beyond measure that instructions given now six weeks ago are now to be acted on,' he confided in October 1848.[28] Equally, he was obliged to acknowledge the uncertain status of regulations. When asked by the authorities in Marylebone whether they had the right to break down doors in the course of nuisance removal Chadwick meekly responded that 'we must have a law officer's opinion'.[29]

Gulson seemed just as confused. Studying the new legislation, he appealed to Chadwick: 'in Corporate towns, like Exeter and Plymouth, which are under Local Act as regards the relief to the poor, who are the authorities upon whom the carrying out your regulations will devolve?'[30] The same applied for Devonport and Bristol. As a further complication, local Boards of Health formed voluntarily escaped the obligations incurred by those compelled into existence. Even so senior an Assistant Commissioner as Gulson recognised that his influence in such a legal morass was limited; in any case, his west of England district contained fifty-eight Boards of Guardians and no inspector could be everywhere at once.

The Devonport Board of Health summarised the basic conflict of interest at play: on the one hand, given the conditions in most of Britain's towns and cities, Parliament sanctioned a better safeguard for the health of the population, while on the other, 'in this country, where the rights of property are so jealously guarded, it may be difficult to legislate'.[31] The outcome was the political compromise of 1848 whereby central government officials communicated with but exercised no clearly defined jurisdiction over varied local government structures, all themselves stipulated by Parliament in Local Acts, the Poor Law Amendment Act or the Municipal Corporations Act.

There was an essentially practical consideration too, as Chadwick was reminded by his political chief: Acts of Parliament might say what they liked but was prosecution for even serious breaches ever a realistic option? Those who served on Boards of Guardians did so voluntarily and for no remuneration. If Guardians felt vulnerable to legal actions, 'they would throw up their appointments ... Would not great confusion be the consequence?' [32] Parliament's acknowledgement that central authority might meddle in what were regarded as essentially local affairs was therefore at best grudging and in consequence the General Board of Health endured a precarious existence. Its five-year term was extended in 1853 but was not renewed again in 1858 when its functions were absorbed into the duties of the Privy Council.

In truth, although cholera in 1849 exposed the inadequacy of the existing legislative framework the age of significant advance in the field of public health still lay well in the future. In the 1850s London and many provincial cities appointed medical officers of health, albeit part-time and untenured, and a new Public Health Act in 1858 conferred upon local authorities the right of compulsory purchase and an increased role in planning and building regulations. The 1858 Act also gave the Privy Council authority over the mortgages which local government bodies needed when raising capital for public works and its medical department thereby became the inspecting body for either sanctioning or refusing applications, effectively giving central government a measure of financial control over local authorities for the first time. Additional Nuisance Removal Acts in 1855, 1860 and 1863 closed off many legal loopholes by which the provisions of their predecessors had been evaded. Sewage purification before discharge into rivers was required under Acts of 1861 and 1865. In 1871 most aspects of local government were brought under the supervision of a Minister in London exercising responsibility as President of the Local Government Board. Two further Public Health Acts of 1872 and 1875 consolidated earlier legislation and provided a legal framework for statutory bodies which lasted until 1936.

By the 1870s most British cities had a wholesome water supply and had undertaken extensive programmes for drainage and sewerage. By the 1870s, too, around 700 towns had established permanent Boards of Health as hostility to the provisions of Westminster legislation began slowly but gradually to diminish. The same decade saw the first effective Food and Drugs legislation while an Act of 1885 began the task of banning pigsties, dairies and cowsheds from urban areas. Generic legislation doubtless raised public expectation but at local level individual initiative and sustained pressure from reforming groups usually remained the driving forces for change. In the naval towns of Devon public health awareness was also clearly enhanced by the role which the Royal Navy played in handling the 1849 crisis.

At the forefront of campaigning and of exposing the inadequate response of many of those responsible for meeting the epidemic was the imposing figure of Nicolas at the Royal Naval Hospital. He badgered Boards of Health into action, he sent out medical staff from the hospital to investigate, to help with public health measures and to treat the sick, and he instigated the litigation which so embarrassed the East Stonehouse Guardians. The Devonport Board of Health paid fulsome tribute to Nicolas's work within its area of jurisdiction as well as to his efforts in East Stonehouse. To Nicolas, its chairman recorded in October 1849, 'the public owe a deep debt of gratitude'. He had proved ever ready 'to meet wants that could not otherwise have been supplied'.[33] Nicolas was a showman who relished the applause which his involvement in civic politics provided. Holding the stage at an enquiry and at the Petty Sessions in the town hall was meat and drink to a man who seemed to thrive on conflict and who wished to project to all around him the image of a fearless captain honour bound at whatever cost to defend what was right for the naval service and for those whose lives were entrusted to his care. To that extent he reflected the Navy's natural concern both for the seafaring populations of Plymouth, Devonport and East Stonehouse as well as for the inmates of his hospital. The latter were surrounded, he judged, by the putrefying and noxious evidence of a local authority negligent in its legal duties. If cholera could not be contained among the sailors and marines of the three towns then the hospital would be overwhelmed with victims and quickly rendered dysfunctional.

Yet there was more to Nicolas's ambition, as those who were obliged to work closely with him soon came to realise. As Nicolas concerned himself increasingly with political matters so his relationship with the medical staff at the Royal Naval Hospital deteriorated. McClure, of course, had no cause for complaint but in that respect he was exceptional. His work with Milroy and the Boards of Health provided exciting and unusual opportunities for a young assistant-surgeon and they gave him the chance to report to and impress both senior naval officers and the Director-General of the medical service. Alone in fact among the hospital's medics, McClure seemed able to work harmoniously with the Captain Superintendent and proved to be an able and convincing adjunct when it came to gathering statistics and medical intelligence. McClure was the one man on the staff whom Nicolas fully trusted and McClure reciprocated with an obvious respect for the Commodore's interest in public health and his zest for getting things done. It was a relationship which earned him the jibe of being Nicolas's 'toady' within the institution as divisions there intensified in the course of the summer of 1849.[34]

The principal rift within the hospital developed between Nicolas and Rae. As medical Inspector it was Rae's task to provide for the patients, which could not be done if his junior colleagues were being despatched all around the towns and nearby villages at the Governor's whim. Infuriating as Bowden's absences in June and July were, Rae could scarcely protest too much since they were at the bidding of Burnett in London. But McClure's repeated absences from hospital duties led to furious exchanges between Rae and Nicolas in July and August and by the height of the epidemic the two men were at daggers drawn. Rae warned Burnett not to be deceived by Nicolas's pompous concern with the poor of the naval towns and his sudden conversion to the cause of public health. Nicolas was playing for all the publicity he could get in order to draw the Board of Admiralty's attention to his devotion to duty and administrative prowess. 'He is working for a name for himself with the powers that be – no matter who suffers,' Rae warned his old friend. '*Self*, *Self*, is the only motive, depend upon it.'[35]

Rae was right about Nicolas's frustrated ambition. It was common knowledge that Nicolas regarded his posting to the hospital and victualling yard in 1847 as but a substitute for what he had really wanted: command at the Devonport dockyard. By 1849 he wanted away from East Stonehouse and to fill a vacancy on the Board of Admiralty. That, however, was never likely. Nicolas's reputation as a headstrong colleague had long gone before him and as his row with Rae became still more embittered during the autumn and winter of 1849 he began to seem temperamentally unstable and obsessed with the trivia of everyday professional disagreements. In the end the Admiralty was obliged to conduct an enquiry into the governance of the Royal Naval Hospital and in February 1850 Nicolas resigned his post. Rae interpreted this outcome as a vindication of his stance all along that Nicolas's involvement in affairs outside the hospital had imposed an unreasonable burden on the medical staff during a period of unprecedented pressure, particularly upon himself and Allen, and that the proper workings of the institution had thereby been compromised and lives put at risk by Nicolas's pursuit of career interest and his unwarranted use of McClure to assist him. Blinded by his own dislike, though, Rae took too narrow a view of Nicolas's duties. The Captain-Superintendent was not there just to provide a chain of command and administrative order conducive to the well-being and wishes of the hospital's surgeons. Whatever his ultimate motivation might have been, it was also Nicolas's job to help to maintain the Navy's standing in an important naval centre.

Whether for its past role in municipal politics, its economic clout in the towns, or the deference which naval officers sometimes arrogantly felt was due them from the citizenry among whom they lived, the Navy was always open to hostility from some who resented its privileges. Maintaining good relations with local dignitaries was therefore part of the work of senior officers who held positions of command in any port or dockyard town. While Rae viewed the hospital through the eyes of a senior surgeon and medical administrator, Nicolas saw it as an important naval foundation dominating East Stonehouse and the Stonehouse Lane area of western Plymouth. But with admissions largely restricted to serving sailors and marines, Nicolas knew that not all the residents of its environs shared his pride in its exclusive status – as indeed one angry letter in the press made plain in August 1849. With the three towns suffering so much from the ravages of cholera, why did their poor have to rely on the scant facilities afforded by temporary wooden and canvas cholera hospitals when one of the nation's leading establishments had a huge capacity which might in the current emergency be given over to the needs of the civilian population? The rooms and space at the Royal Naval Hospital were public property and the sick of the towns should be taken there; why were 40,000 or 50,000 needy inhabitants in the naval towns considered any less Her Majesty's subjects at this time of crisis than 4,000 or 5,000 sailors? [36]

Set in this context, Nicolas's anxiety to be seen to be helping the towns' cholera hospitals with stores and provisions, both from the naval hospital and from the victualling yard, his use of the eager McClure, his litigation via the Admiralty solicitors and his high-profile campaigning for greater action by the local Boards of Health served a purpose to which Rae appeared oblivious and for which even the Board of Admiralty ultimately displayed little gratitude. If meddling in matters beyond the walls of the Royal Naval Hospital was then influenced further by his personal ambition, Nicolas was not the only senior figure in naval service against whom that charge could be laid. Burnett, whose patented chloride of zinc was adopted by the Royal Navy in 1851 amid verifiable claims that the Treasury would be saved £200,000 annually,[37] also showed no hesitation in depriving Rae of much-needed assistance when Bowden was sent to conduct the extraordinary experiment at Noss in July 1849 by which Burnett hoped to establish once and for all the efficacy of his disinfecting and antiseptic fluid. Like Nicolas, Burnett could be adept at cloaking his own aspirations in efforts to advance the common good.

Even so, individual experimentation was not uncommon in public health work and, business interests aside, Burnett's enthusiasm for epidemiology was no less than might have been expected from a man of science in his position. Inspectors from the General Board of Health certainly saw themselves in this light. Sutherland, for one, took the opportunity which arose in Dumfries at the end of 1848: 'it enabled us to try the most complete preventive experiment I believe on record', he reflected.[38] Not only did Sutherland claim credit for stamping out cholera in Dumfries but he asserted that his experimental methods had been so successful that the parochial authorities in Glasgow had subsequently agreed to apply them to the city's 300,000 inhabitants. Sutherland indeed relished his role at the forefront of investigation and epidemic control and sounded even wistful as the crisis abated. 'Our measures were just beginning to be understood when the cholera disappeared,' he mused; a great chance for the advancement of scientific knowledge and his own prominence was thus slipping away.[39]

Yet if concern for the sick was tempered by career advantage or the prospect of commercial gain, for those who benefited thereby the mixture of motives was, of course, largely irrelevant. The chloride was used plentifully on the houses of the sick at Torpoint in September, and in both the St Germans and Plympton St Mary Unions the expressions of gratitude to the Navy for the assistance rendered were profuse and sincere. Although Bowden could never quite produce the scientific proof of effectiveness which Burnett wanted for his patent most agreed that his efforts to tame the epidemic in Noss had been remarkably successful. Back in Plymouth, McClure demonstrated a more persuasive methodology, but such proof as Burnett needed would inevitably be illusory until the precise nature of cholera itself was known.

Nevertheless, medical opinion and public health reformers alike had long drawn the obvious conclusion that whatever the exact cause of cholera and other epidemic diseases, environmental squalor, slum accommodation and the poverty and ignorance of so large a proportion of the nation's population were all evils which needed redress if Britain was ever to be free from such threats; in Plymouth, along with many other cities, the experience of 1849 drove a growing debate about the worth of traditional local government structures and the benefits which could follow from change. In Plymouth, typically, this debate focused on whether the provisions of the 1848 Public Health Act should be adopted whereby a permanently constituted Board of Health, answerable to the General Board in London, would take over statutory responsibility for a proper water supply, sewerage, refuse removal and, by employing medical officers, would oversee all matters pertaining to public health. Authority to raise a rate for these purposes and even to borrow money for structural projects would also be transferred. The initiative for such change was unlikely to come from Improvement Commissioners, which was why the 1848 Act had stipulated that if a two-thirds majority and at least 10 per cent of ratepayers petitioned for adopting the Act then inspectors would be sent from London to investigate and advise.[40] By the end of 1853, however, only 164 towns had completed the protracted process.[41]

Some campaigners in Plymouth had argued that the permanent mechanism offered by the Public Health Act should be adopted even in 1849. For reformers, the ineffectiveness which they believed characterised the voluntary Boards of Health during the cholera emergency was all the evidence needed for the benefits which would accrue. Proposals and rebuttals appeared in the press from September 1849 onwards and in December a special meeting of Plymouth's Improvement Commissioners was called in order to consider their response. By that time one-tenth of the ratepayers had got up a petition in favour of change and a number of private residents had already memorialised the General Board of Health for an inspector to be sent.[42] But the Improvement Commissioners voted against any alteration. Central to the opposition was not a belief that its local government structures had served the citizens of the town with great distinction during their tribulations in 1849 but rather the simple conviction that those men who comprised them were at least Plymouth men who ultimately had more interest in the welfare of the population than distant officials making rules for places which they may never even have visited.

Momentum for reform might have been greater had not Latimer rather surprisingly shared this reservation. For all his progressive instincts, he was proud of his city and its individual character; he even mellowed sufficiently over the years to be elected mayor in 1871. In October 1849 the *Journal* cautioned that 'our Local Act is well understood by all and works most efficiently'. Referring to the sewers and drains of Plymouth, it concluded that 'nothing is gained by transferring these duties to the Town Council as the Board of Health – for what guarantee have we that greater efforts will be made by these functionaries than are actually making at present by the Commissioners?'[43] New Local Acts for Plymouth were proposed as a means of fending off those who lobbied for change and the high costs which the Borough would incur in legal fees were repeatedly stressed. The Guardians of the Plymouth Union were even accused of publishing false statistics on pauperism in order to confuse the ratepayers. Morrish, a long-standing advocate of reform, claimed that although the Guardians said the number of paupers had doubled in the decade after 1841, this was at variance with data published by the Poor Law Board. The Guardians would have the population believe that the rapidly increasing numbers claiming relief were swamping them. Morrish, by contrast, having long seen his colleagues at work, asserted that their shortcomings were more properly attributed to 'the inadaption of the present constitution of the Plymouth Guardians to the times in which we live, their faulty administration of the law and the want of a superior controlling power'. Gulson certainly agreed, but even three years after the epidemic it was still the old familiar story. The Poor Law Board was 'fully aware that the administration at Plymouth is faulty and requires alteration', he minuted. However, as always, it had 'very limited powers in this respect'.[44]

Yet the reformers could not be kept quiet and no sooner had the cholera passed than the Guardians faced more questions, this time concerning their pitiful attempts to address the problem of building a new workhouse. A meeting called to consider plans was inquorate on 2 January 1850 and two further meetings on 11 January and 20 March postponed a decision further 'in consequence of the heavy expense on the ratepayers occasioned by the late visitation of the cholera'.[45] Then came the annual elections in May, following which the Guardians announced that legal advice would have to be sought before any decision could be reached. A workhouse committee was set up with the trusty Beer as chairman, but by September even he had progressed no further than writing to enquire of the Poor Law Board how the money necessary for construction might be raised.

To the disappointment of the more frugally minded Plymouth Guardians there was a prompt reply from London: the Guardians were authorised both to borrow a large sum repayable over twenty years and to sell the old site once the new building was opened. Since all plans for new workhouses had to be approved by the Poor Law Board the option of an inadequate and hence inexpensive edifice was closed; the Guardians finally seemed to have been manoeuvred into a position where a large development had to begin. But help came unexpectedly from their neighbours in Devonport, where the same process was under way but where, when construction tenders had been invited, all the returns exceeded the approved budget. Everything in Devonport had been suspended for six months and the Guardians in Plymouth immediately seized upon this opportunity to procrastinate. Fired by a common desire to save money, the Plymouth and Stoke Damerel Guardians investigated the possibility of merging their Unions, thereby requiring only one workhouse. Predictably, nothing came of so desperate a proposal but there remained a last trick to play: obliged to draw up a building plan, the Plymouth Guardians turned to acclaimed experts in delay and insensitivity to hostile opinion: their counterparts in East Stonehouse. There they engaged as their architect Charles Chapple, the former chairman of the East Stonehouse Board of Health and still a prominent Poor Law Guardian of the parish.

Chapple corresponded with the Poor Law Board about his design. A building to accommodate up to 600 inmates was envisaged with apartments for the workhouse officers and other facilities, all of which took time to finalise. In January 1851 Chapple asked for more advice about how lunatic paupers were to be housed and then, when advised that separate quarters would be needed, proceeded to submit drawings in July which conspicuously failed to meet the specifications. At this point the process of tendering threw the project into near terminal confusion since only three bids were within the £10,000 borrowing limit stipulated by the Poor Law Board and from these Chapple recommended one which he knew had no chance of approval, lacking as it did a chapel, a dining area and sufficient height and ventilation in the rooms. Arguments about new workhouses in both Plymouth and Devonport dragged on for a further three years.[46] The Guardians showed remarkable tenacity both in asserting their autonomy and in minimising charges to the ratepayers who elected them to office. Unwittingly they also demonstrated to a growing number of local government reformers precisely those wrongs and influences to offset which the benign force of central government was invoked and which gave ever greater credibility to the groundswell of argument in favour of change.

Matters were brought to a head in 1851 when the General Board of Health ordered an investigation into the health and sanitation of Plymouth. When evidence was gathered in January 1852 Plymouth, like Devonport and East Stonehouse, was confirmed as having a death rate averaged over seven years above the threshold of twenty-three per thousand, and the superintending inspector, Robert Rawlinson, had no hesitation in judging the town to be among the most unhealthy in Britain. Rawlinson, however, was not as harsh on the old local government structures as some might have hoped. Although the Improvement Commissioners had remained the butt of sustained criticism since 1849 he gave them credit for expenditure on street widening, pavement improvements and constructing new sewers in different locations. Their failing lay in the fact that these works were unco-ordinated and that Plymouth's overall deficiencies in drainage and sewerage simply could not be addressed by a body whose remit and revenue raising capacity were so restricted. Given that Gibson, the leading Commissioner, now presided over the Town Council as mayor of Plymouth, this conciliatory tone would have avoided much ill feeling, though Rawlinson's conclusions were emphatic. Published at the beginning of 1853, his report recommended that the provisions of the 1848 Public Health Act be applied and that one elected authority thereby should have control. He had, he added, conducted similar enquiries in other towns; yet 'in none have I found local improvement more required'.[47]

In the same year more than 5,000 inhabitants petitioned against further Local Acts for Plymouth and with Rawlinson's report to guide reformers the fate of the old structures with their divided responsibilities for health and sanitation was effectively sealed. In 1854, and with only muted dissent, the Improvement Commissioners were abolished and a permanent Board of Health formed by the mayor, aldermen and burgesses of the borough.[48] The Town Council therefore acquired the statutory powers which came with the 1848 Act and which soon enabled work to begin on an entirely new sewerage system for Plymouth, made possible in part because future rate revenue could henceforth be mortgaged as security for loans. Slum quarters were also demolished in the years ahead and by 1860 the Plymouth Board of Health had refurbished the public baths and wash-houses, reviewed the state of slaughterhouses and the locations of other offensive trades, removed many of the nuisances which so despoiled streets and public spaces and even taken under its administration public parks for the recreation of the citizenry.

Of course, not all improvements after 1849 required new law. The old Commissioners had not always lacked sufficient powers; it was often the will to use them which had been missing when compromised by self-interest or when broader political opposition or that from individuals determined to uphold ancient rights made the costs and effort not worthwhile. Nor, manifestly, did antipathy towards central government intrusion evaporate in 1849. The importance of cholera lay in its stark revelation of the danger of neglecting public health – not in its weakening of civic identity. The naval towns of Devon highlight the forces ranged for and against local government reform and showed how failings, real and perceived, among the established authorities could alter the balance of argument and undermine the case of those who urged that local interests were still best served by a preservation of the status quo. The scale of the 1849 epidemic in Plymouth, Devonport and East Stonehouse could have overwhelmed any structures in place and the response within each town inevitably would owe much to the commitment of individual dignitaries as well as to the constitutional composition of whatever bodies they sat upon. In the 1840s and beyond, embracing the instruments of change was no guarantee that improvement would occur: adopting the 1848 Act, for example, allowed Plymouth to appoint a medical officer of health but none was in post until 1890. To stress that, however, would belittle other achievements. The events of 1849 established a clear direction for change, slow as the pace at times might seem. The suffering, confusion and recrimination which accompanied the cholera epidemic as it swept through the three towns proved sufficient to ensure that their politics in future would never be the same.

Notes

Introduction

1. Specifically T. McKeown, *The Modern Rise of Population* (London, 1976). The ensuing academic controversy is revisited in S. Szreter, 'The Importance of Social Intervention in Britain's Mortality Decline *c.* 1850–1914: A Re-interpretation of the Role of Public Health', *Social History of Medicine*, 1 (1988), pp. 1–37.
2. See P. Thane (ed.), *The Origins of British Social Policy* (London, 1978), p. 11.
3. For the debate regarding the pace of change see G. Kearns, *Aspects of Cholera, Society end Space in Nineteenth-century England and Wales* (University of Cambridge, PhD thesis, 1985), pp. 286–303.
4. Discussion of the interaction of nineteenth-century epidemics with social and cultural values is contained in C. E. Rosenberg, 'Cholera in Nineteenth-century Europe: A Tool for Social and Economic Analysis', in C. E. Rosenberg (ed.), *Explaining Epidemics and Other Studies in the History of Medicine* (Cambridge, 1992), pp. 109–121.
5. K. Wrightson, 'The Social Order of Early Modern England: Three Approaches', in L. Bonfield, R. M. Smith and K. Wrightson (eds), *The World We Have Gained: Histories of Population and Social Structure* (Oxford, 1986), p. 202. The worth of local studies is also analysed in G. Kearns, 'Cholera and Public Health Reform in Nineteenth-century England and Wales: Interpreting the Geographical Patterns', *The Society for the Social History of Medicine*, 35 (1984), pp. 30–2.
6. J. V. Pickstone, 'Medicine in Industrial Britain: The Uses of Local Studies', *Social History of Medicine*, 2 (1989), pp. 197–203. The work reviewed is H. Marland, *Medicine and Society in Wakefield and Huddersfield, 1780–1870* (Cambridge, 1987).

1: Disease, Politics and Poverty in Nineteenth-century Britain

1. An extensive bibliography exists regarding cholera in the nineteenth

century. Among the most authoritative works are M. Pelling, *Cholera, Fever and English Medicine 1825–1865* (Oxford, 1978); R. J. Evans, *Death in Hamburg: Society and politics in the Cholera Years 1830–1910* (Oxford, 1987); and A. Hardy, 'Cholera, Quarantine and the English Preventive System, 1850–1895', *Medical History*, 37 (1993), pp. 250–69.

2. J. Snow, *On the Mode of Communication of Cholera* (London, 1849).
3. Public health reform in the context of such widespread change in British society is comprehensively covered in F. B. Smith, *The People's Health 1830–1910* (London, 1979); and A. S. Wohl, *Endangered Lives: Public Health in Victorian Britain* (London, 1983). Older, though valuable, is W. M. Frazer, *A History of English Public Health 1834–1939* (London, 1950).
4. Statistics regarding the impact of disease upon the population are from Wohl, op. cit., pp. 128–33; and Smith, op. cit., p. 288. See also S. Szreter, 'The Importance of Social Intervention', pp. 11 and 13; and R. J. Morris, *Cholera 1832: The Social Response to an Epidemic* (London, 1976), p. 12. The most thorough research in this area from the 1850s onwards is produced in A. Hardy, *The Epidemic Streets: Infectious Disease and the Rise of Preventive Medicine, 1856–1900* (Oxford, 1993); and A. Hardy, 'Smallpox in London: Factors in the Decline of Disease in the Nineteenth Century', *Medical History*, 27 (1983), pp. 111–38.
5. Medical remedies are analysed in N. Howard-Jones, 'Cholera Therapy in the Nineteenth Century', *Journal of the History of Medicine and Allied Sciences*, 27 (1972), pp. 373–95.
6. A point explained in G. Kearns, *Urban Epidemics and Historical Geography: Cholera in London, 1848–9* (Norwich, 1985), pp. 16–18.
7. *The Plymouth and Devonport Weekly Journal* (hereafter *The Journal*), 15 February 1849, p. 7.
8. Chadwick's life and work is most recently and authoritatively analysed in C. Hamlin, *Public Health and Social Justice in the Age of Chadwick: Britain, 1800–1854* (Cambridge, 1998). Earlier biographical works, however, remain valuable sources, specifically S. E. Finer, *The Life and Times of Sir Edwin Chadwick* (London, 1952); R. A. Lewis, *Edwin Chadwick and the Public Health Movement 1832–1854* (London, 1952); M. W. Flinn (ed.) *Report on the Sanitary Condition of the Labouring Population of Great Britain 1842 by Edwin Chadwick* (Edinburgh, 1965); R. Klein, 'Edwin Chadwick 1800–1890', in P. Barker (ed.), *Founders of the Welfare State* (London, 1984), pp. 8–16;

and D. Gladstone (ed.), *Pioneers in Social Welfare III: Edwin Chadwick: Nineteenth-century Social Reformer* (London, 1997).

9. Farr's particular contribution to public health reform is discussed in J. M. Eyler, *Victorian Social Medicine: The Ideas and Methods of William Farr* (Baltimore, 1979); and L. Goldman, 'Statistics and the Science of Society in Early Victorian Britain: An Intellectual Context for the General Register Office', *Social History of Medicine*, 4 (1991), pp. 415–34. See also S. Szreter, 'The G. R. O. and the Public Health Movement in Britain, 1837–1914', *Social History of Medicine*, 4 (1991), pp. 435–63; and J. M. Eyler, 'William Farr on the Cholera: The Sanitarian's Disease Theory and the Statistician's Method', *Journal of the History of Medicine and Allied Sciences*, 28 (1973), pp. 79–100.
10. R. G. Paterson, 'The Health of Towns Association in Great Britain 1844–1849', *Bulletin of the History of Medicine*, 22 (1948), pp. 373–402.
11. Chadwick to Burton, 29 September 1849, *Papers of John Hill Burton*, National Library of Scotland, Edinburgh, MS 9406.
12. The work of the early years of the Board was evaluated in a preliminary *Report by the General Board of Health on the Measures Adopted for the Execution of the Nuisance Removal and Diseases Prevention Act and the Public Health Act up to July 1849*, Parliamentary Accounts and Papers, XXIV (1849); and more fully in *Report of the General Board of Health on the Administration of the Public Health Act and the Nuisances Removal and Diseases Prevention Acts from 1848 to 1854*, P.P. XXXV (1854).
13. Carlisle to Russell, 23 September 1849, *Papers of Lord John Russell*, Public Record Office, London, PRO 30/22/8A.
14. B. Keith-Lucas, *The Unreformed Local Government System* (London, 1980), p. 18.
15. Local government reform in the mid-nineteenth century supports a huge bibliography, although it can be well understood from R. J. Morris, *Class, Sect and Party: The Making of the British Middle Class, Leeds 1820–1850* (Manchester, 1990); D. Fraser, *Power and Authority in the Victorian City* (Oxford, 1979); D. Fraser, *Urban Politics in Victorian England: The Structures of Politics in Victorian Cities* (Leicester, 1976); B. Keith-Lucas, *English Local Government in the Nineteenth and Twentieth Centuries* (London, 1977); and E. P. Hennock, *Fit and Proper Persons: Ideal and Reality in Nineteenth-century Urban Government* (London, 1973). See too D. Fraser (ed.), *Municipal Reform and the Industrial City* (Leicester, 1982).
16. A. Alexander, *Borough Government and Politics: Reading 1835–1985* (London, 1985), p. 6.

17. Hennock, op. cit., p. 180.
18. Ebrington to Russell, 10 January 1836, *Russell Papers*, PRO 30/22/2A.
19. Fraser, *Urban Politics in Victorian England*, p. 91.
20. Alexander, op. cit., p. 3.
21. N. C. Edsall, 'Varieties of Radicalism: Attwood, Cobden and the Local Politics of Municipal Incorporation', *Historical Journal*, 16 (1973), pp. 93–4.
22. Fraser (ed.), *Municipal Reform and the Industrial City*, p. 6.
23. Wohl, op. cit., p. 166.
24. Hennock, op. cit., p. 186 fn.
25. For further information concerning the peculiarities of Leeds, Birmingham, Liverpool and Bradford see Hennock, op. cit., pp. 182–3, 191; and A. Elliott, 'Municipal Government in Bradford in the Mid-Nineteenth Century', in Fraser (ed.), *Municipal Reform and the Industrial City*, pp. 112–61.
26. Chadwick to Ashley, 11 May 1844, 2181 (2), and Chadwick to Morpeth, 21 July 1848, 1055, *Papers of Sir Edwin Chadwick*, University College, London.
27. Among the best studies of mid-nineteenth-century Poor Law reform are F. Driver, *Power and Pauperism: The Workhouse System, 1834–1884* (Cambridge, 1993); L. H. Lees, 'The Survival of the Unfit: Welfare Policies and Family Maintenance in Nineteenth-century London', in P. Mandler (ed.), *The Uses of Charity: The Poor on Relief in the Nineteenth-century Metropolis* (Philadelphia, 1990), pp. 68–91; A. Digby, *The Poor Law in Nineteenth-century England and Wales* (London, 1982); U. Henriques, *Before the Welfare State: Social Administration in Early Industrial Britain* (London, 1979); J. H. Treble, *Urban Poverty in Britain 1830–1914* (London, 1979); M. E. Rose, *The Relief of Poverty, 1834–1914* (London, 1972); D. Roberts, *Victorian Origins of the British Welfare State* (New Haven, 1960); D. Fraser, *The Evolution of the British Welfare State: A History of Social Policy Since the Industrial Revolution* (London, 1973).
28. J. D. Marshall, *The Old Poor Law 1795–1834* (London, 1968), pp. 23, 26–7; M. E. Rose, *The English Poor Law 1780–1930* (Newton Abbot, 1971), pp. 40–1. The Poor Rate in England and Wales quadrupled between 1790 and 1820. See D. Englander, *Poverty and Poor Law Reform in Britain: From Chadwick to Booth, 1834–1914* (London, 1998), p. 3.
29. Keith-Lucas, *The Unreformed Local Government System*, p. 76.
30. Gulson to Chadwick, 4 October 1848, *Chadwick Papers*, 907.

31. Chadwick to Russell, 27 July 1838, *Russell Papers*, PRO 30/22/3B.
32. Petition to Poor Law Commissioners, 18 December 1847, Ministry of Health Records, PRO London, MH 19/178.
33. Memorandum by Gulson, 23 September 1850, MH 19/178.
34. Fraser, *Urban Politics in Victorian England*, p. 71. See also Rose, *The English Poor Law*, pp. 135–7.
35. Driver, *Power and Pauperism*, p. 35; and A. Digby, 'The Rural Poor Law', in D. Fraser (ed.), *The New Poor Law in the Nineteenth Century* (London, 1976), p. 157.
36. Digby, *The Poor Law in Nineteenth-century England and Wales*, p. 16. Workhouses are analysed in great detail in M. A. Crowther, *The Workhouse System 1834–1929: The History of an English Social Institution* (London, 1981); and R. Hodgkinson, *The Origins of the National Health Service: The Medical Services of the New Poor Law, 1834–1871* (London, 1967), pp. 147–75.
37. Digby, 'The Rural Poor Law', in Fraser (ed.), *The New Poor Law in the Nineteenth Century* p. 154.
38. Gulson to Chadwick, 5 July 1836, *Chadwick Papers*, 907.
39. Memorandum by Gulson, 23 September 1850, MH 19/178.
40. Digby, *The Poor Law in Nineteenth-century England and Wales*, p. 23; and Rose, *The Relief of Poverty*, pp. 17, 19.
41. Official figures for expenditure and the numbers of paupers relieved between 1840 and 1847 are from the *Fourteenth Report of the Poor Law Commissioners*, P.P. XXXIII (1847–48), and conveniently reproduced in Rose, *The English Poor Law*, pp. 128–9. Copious compilations as to the numbers relieved and the costs in the subsequent two years are to be found in the *Report of the Commissioners for Administering the laws for Relief of the poor in England 1848*, P.P. XXV (1849); and *Second Annual Report of the Poor Law Board 1849*, P.P. XXVII (1850).
42. Gulson to Buller, 10 April 1848, MH 32/29.
43. *Reports to the Poor Law Board on the Laws of Settlement, and Removal of the Poor*, P.P. XXVII (1850). The complexities of settlement are discussed in and these figures are from M. E. Rose, 'Settlement, Removal and the New Poor Law', in Fraser (ed.), *The New Poor Law in the Nineteenth Century*, pp. 25–44; and Rose, *The English Poor Law*, pp. 191–4. See also Englander, op. cit., p. 15; and an excellent study by D. Ashforth, 'Settlement and Removal in Urban Areas: Bradford, 1834–71', in M. E. Rose (ed.), *The Poor and the City: The English Poor Law in Its Urban Context, 1834–1914* (Leicester, 1985), pp. 58–91.

44. Gulson to Poor Law Commissioners, 23 February 1847, MH 32/29.
45. D. Ashforth, 'The Urban Poor Law', in Fraser (ed.), *The New Poor Law in the Nineteenth Century*, p. 146; and Ashforth, 'Settlement and Removal in Urban Areas', in Rose (ed.), *The Poor and the City*, p. 79.
46. The *Journal*, 15 March 1849, p. 3.
47. Memorandum by Nicholls, 18 November 1850, MH 19/178; and Chadwick to Bracebridge, 22 March 1847, *Chadwick Papers*, 2181 (20).
48. Baines to Russell, 11 October 1851, *Russell Papers*, PRO 30/22/9G (l).
49. Chadwick to Russell, 5 December 1848, *Chadwick Papers*, 1733.
50. Hennock, op. cit., p. 5; and Elliott, op. cit., p. 117.
51. Alexander, op. cit., p. 30.
52. Lewis, op. cit., pp. 301–18, cites this case and analyses the effectiveness of local Boards of Health.
53. Morpeth to Chadwick, 21 February 1848, *Chadwick Papers*, 1055.
54. Carlisle to Russell, 3 August 1849, *Russell Papers*, PRO 30/22/8A.
55. Chadwick to Ebrington, 13 October 1848, *Chadwick Papers*, 755.
56. Austin to the Clerks of Union Guardians, 15 August 1849, MH 10/100.
57. These statistics are from Wohl, op. cit., pp. 84, 89–90, 95, 111; Smith, op. cit., pp. 197–8; and Alexander, op. cit., p. 19.
58. The expansion of professional and scientific expertise in early-nineteenth-century Britain is analysed in C. Hamlin, *A Science of Impurity: Water Analysis in Nineteenth-century Britain* (Bristol, 1990); R. MacLeod (ed.), *Government and Expertise: Specialists, Administrators and Professionals, 1860–1919* (Cambridge, 1988); and A. J. Youngson, *The Scientific Revolution in Victorian Medicine* (London, 1979).
59. The rise of the medical profession in the nineteenth century is thoroughly covered in A. Digby, *Making a Medical Living: Doctors and Patients in the English Market for Medicine, 1720–1911* (Cambridge, 1994); I. Waddington, *The Medical Profession in the Industrial Revolution* (Dublin, 1984); M. J. Peterson, *The Medical Profession in Mid-Victorian London* (Berkeley, 1978); N. Parry and J. Parry, *The Rise of the Medical Profession: A Study of Collective Social Mobility* (London, 1976), pp. 104–30; G. Clark, *A History of the Royal College of Physicians of London* (Oxford, 1966); and F.N.L. Poynter (ed.), *The Evolution of Medical Practice in Britain* (London, 1961).
60. Developments in medical education are explored in S.C. Lawrence, *Charitable Knowledge: Hospital Pupils and Practitioners in Eighteenth-*

century London (Cambridge, 1996); and S.C. Lawrence, 'Private Enterprise and Public Interests: Medical Education and the Apothecaries' Act, 1780–1825', in R. French and A. Wear (eds), *British Medicine in an Age of Reform* (London, 1991), pp. 45–73. See also F.N.L. Poynter (ed.), *The Evolution of Medical Education in Britain* (London, 1966); and S. W. F. Holloway, 'Medical Education in England, 1830–1858: A Sociological Analysis', *History*, 49 (1964), pp. 299–324.

61. V. M. Crosse, *A Surgeon in the Early Nineteenth Century: The Life and Times of John Green Crosse, 1790–1850* (London, 1968), p. 40.
62. Guyther to General Board of Health, 17 October 1848, MH 13/245.
63. There is debate about the emergence of general practice, specifically relating to how early in the late eighteenth or early nineteenth centuries the development occurred. The issue is investigated and the overall structure of the medical profession authoritatively revealed in I.S.L. Loudon, *Medical Care and the General Practitioner 1750–1850* (Oxford, 1986). See also I.S.L. Loudon, 'The Concept of the Family Doctor', *Bulletin of the History of Medicine*, 58 (1984), pp. 347–62; Waddington, op. cit., pp. 1–49; and Parry and Parry, op. cit., pp. 104–30. The figures are from Loudon, *Medical Care and the General Practitioner*, pp. 208–27.
64. The Poor Law medical service is thoroughly covered in Loudon, *Medical Care and the General Practitioner*, pp. 228–48; M. W. Flinn, 'Medical Services Under the New Poor Law', in Fraser (ed.), *The New Poor Law in the Nineteenth Century*, pp. 45–66; and most comprehensively in Hodgkinson, *The Origins of the National Health Service.*
65. Gulson to Chadwick, 1836, *Chadwick Papers*, 907.
66. These figures are from Loudon, *Medical Care and the General Practitioner*, pp. 240–2; Flinn, 'Medical Services Under the New Poor Law', in Fraser (ed.), *The New Poor Law in the Nineteenth Century*, p. 51; and Ashforth, 'The Urban Poor Law', in Fraser (ed.), *The New Poor Law in the Nineteenth Century*, p. 140.
67. Petition of the Halifax Union medical officers, April 1849, MH 25/6.
68. See Hamlin, *Public Health and Social Justice*, p. 263; Wohl, op. cit., pp. 180–2; and C. F. Brockington, *Public Health in the Nineteenth Century* (London, 1965), p. 139.
69. Figures are from Loudon, *Medical Care and the General Practitioner*, pp. 238–42, 307; and Lees, op. cit., p. 83.
70. Black to Baines, 5 September 1849, MH 25/6.
71. Sutherland to Chadwick, 30 August 1847, *Chadwick Papers*, 920.
72. Lewis, op. cit., pp. 198, 205.

2: The Boroughs and Unions of South Devon

1. Plymouth's history and development are recorded in C. Gill, *Plymouth: A New History* (London, 1993); C. Robinson, *Victorian Plymouth* (Plymouth, 1991); and J. C. Trewin, *Portrait of Plymouth* (London, 1973). Older, though with much interesting detail, is L. Jewitt, *A History of Plymouth* (London, 1873).
2. The *Journal* first appeared in 1817 and survived until 1860, when relaunched as a daily entitled the *Western Daily Mercury*. Latimer was proprietor of both. Jewitt, op. cit., p. 642.
3. Town Clerks for Plymouth, Devonport and East Stonehouse 1491–1953, Plymouth and West Devon Record Office, Plymouth, 1546/19.
4. The *Journal*, 20 September 1849, p. 8.
5. R. Rawlinson, *Report to the General Board of Health on a Preliminary Enquiry into the Sewerage, Drainage, and Supply of water, and the Sanitary Condition of the Inhabitants of the Borough of Plymouth, in the County of Devon* (London, 1853), p. 17.
6. For the Improvement Commission's annual income 1824–52 and its debt see Rawlinson, *Report to the General Board of Health on Plymouth*, pp. 26–7.
7. The *Journal*, 8 November 1849, p. 6.
8. Deposition of Beard, 11 August 1843, in Weale to Poor Law Board, 2 February 1844, MH 12/2519.
9. Family ties and the role of solicitors in local government are discussed in Keith-Lucas, *The Unreformed Local Government System*, pp. 61, 152–4.
10. Rodd to Poor Law Board, 11 February 1850, MH 12/2223.
11. Fraser, *Urban Politics in Victorian England*, pp. 58–9, 85–90; and Morris, *Class, Sect and Party*, p. 204. See also Rose, *The English Poor Law*, p. 135. The most specific study on this theme is D. Fraser, 'The Poor Law as a Political Institution', in Fraser (ed.), *The New Poor Law in the Nineteenth Century*, pp. 111–27.
12. Clouter to Poor Law Board, 9 February 1850, MH 12/2223.
13. Putt to Poor Law Board, 7 October 1851, MH 12/2422.
14. The *Journal*, 23 August 1849, p. 8.
15. Mortimer to Lumley, 21 November 1851, MH 12/2422.
16. Minute by Gulson, 22 October 1851, on Mortimer to Lumley, 15 October 1851, MH 12/2422.
17. Memorandum by Gulson, 27 November 1849, MH 32/29.

18. Hughes to Poor Law Board, 6 May 1852, MH 12/2422.
19. The finances of the Plymouth Guardians and abuses at the workhouse are conveniently set out in the *Journal*, 1 March 1849, p. 2; and Mortimer to Baines, 21 November 1851, MH 12/2422, although it is not easy to reconcile these with figures cited in the Poor Law Board's reports in P.P. XXV (1849) and P.P. XXVII (1850). The former report gives £17,045 as the sum spent on poor relief in 1848. The corresponding figure for the year to 25 March 1847 in the *Fourteenth Report of the Poor Law Commissioners*, P.P. XXXIII (1847–48), was only £10,474 expended on relieving the poor.
20. Minute by Gulson, 28 April 1849, on Poor Law Board to Arnold, 27 April 1849, MH 12/2223.
21. While scholarship has explored the politics of local democracy in relation to Town Councils after 1835 much less is known about the politicisation of elections for Boards of Guardians, Improvement Commissions and even highway authorities, all of which frequently had greater powers to levy rates. See, however, Fraser, *Urban Politics in Victorian England*, pp. 59–90; Smith, op. cit., p. 361; Morris, *Class, Sect and Party*, pp. 123-4. and Fraser, 'The Poor Law as a Political Institution', in Fraser (ed.), *The New Poor Law in the Nineteenth Century*, pp. 111–27.
22. Expenditure on poor relief is given as £3,655 in East Stonehouse in 1848 in the Poor Law Board report, P.P. XXV (1849). The rate levied amounted to £5,114 and total expenditure from the parish rate was £4,137.
23. The *Journal*, 20 December 1849, p. 3.
24. East Stonehouse Guardians to Poor Law Board, 24 January 1850, MH 12/2223.
25. Ashforth, 'The Urban Poor Law', in Fraser (ed.), *The New Poor Law in the Nineteenth Century*, p. 142; and Fraser, *Urban Politics in Victorian England*, pp. 68–9.
26. East Stonehouse Guardians to Poor Law Board, 24 January 1850, MH 12/2223.
27. Cornish to Poor Law Board, 19 June 1849, MH 12/2223.
28. Poor Law Board report, P.P. XXV (1849). The rate levied in Stoke Damerel in 1848 amounted to £12,530 and the total expenditure from the parish rate was £12,495.
29. The *Journal*, 20 December 1849, p. 8.

30. Mortimer to Lumley, 11 November 1850, MH 12/2422.
31. Memorandum by Gulson, 12 December 1849, MH 12/2422.
32. These figures can be collated from Mortimer to Lumley, 15 October 1851, and Expenditure by the Guardians of the Poor of the Borough of Plymouth for the years ending May 1850 and 1851, MH 12/2422; and Certificate Stating the Numbers of Poor in East Stonehouse, 21 February 1850, MH 12/2223.
33. Gulson to Baines, 22 January 1850. Gulson's economic survey of the West Country is developed further in letters to Baines, 12 March and 12 June 1849, also in MH 32/29.

3: Naval Towns and Naval Medicine

1. The *Journal*, 5 July 1849, p. 2.
2. Tenth Annual Report, 4 February 1850, Records of the South Devon and East Cornwall Hospital, Plymouth and West Devon Record Office, Annual Reports 1840–50, 709/1.
3. Minute, 16 March 1849, Records of the Grey School, Plymouth and West Devon Record Office, Minutes of Trustees and Committee 1843–55, 423/3/6.
4. Tenth Annual Report, 4 February 1850, 709/1. The hospital's expansion in the 1840s is also explained in Gill, op. cit., p. 231; and the *Journal*, 8 February 1849, p. 6. Details regarding the Plymouth Royal Eye Infirmary are in the *Journal*, 11 January 1849, p. 2; and the *Journal*, 28 June 1849, p. 1.
5. Loudon, *Medical Care and the General Practitioner*, p. 306.
6. K.A.Webb, '*One of the Most Useful Charities in the City': York Dispensary 1788–1988* (York, 1988) pp. 3, 7.
7. S. T. Anning, 'A History of Medicine in Leeds', *Proceedings of the Leeds Philosophical and Literary Society, Literary and Historical Section*, 16 (1978), p. 215.
8. There are specific studies of the importance of public dispensaries by I. Loudon, 'The Origins and Growth of the Dispensary Movement in England', *Bulletin of the History of Medicine*, 55 (1981), pp. 322–42; B. Croxson, 'The Public and Private Faces of Eighteenth-century London Dispensary Charity', *Medical History*, 41 (1997), 127–49; R. Kilpatrick, 'Living in the Light': Dispensaries, Philanthropy and Medical Reform in Late Eighteenth-century London', in A. Cunningham and R. French (eds), *The Medical Enlightenment of the*

Eighteenth Century (Cambridge, 1990), pp. 254–80; and Hodgkinson, *The Origins of the National Health Service*, pp. 205–13. Outside London the Dispensary movement is analysed in J. V. Pickstone, *Medicine and Industrial Society: A History of Hospital Development in Manchester and Its Region, 1752–1946* (Manchester, 1985), pp. 64–75; H. Marland, 'Lay and Medical Conceptions of Medical Charity During the Nineteenth Century: The Case of the Huddersfield General Dispensary and Infirmary', in J. Barry and C. Jones (eds), *Medicine and Charity Before the Welfare State* (London, 1991), pp. 149–71; M. Railton, *Early Medical Services: Berkshire and South Oxfordshire from 1740* (Chippenham, 1994), pp. 21–9; C. B. Perry, *The Voluntary Medical Institutions of Bristol* (Bristol, 1984), pp. 7–8; and R. Guest-Gornall, 'The Warrington Dispensary Library', *Medical History*, 11 (1967), pp. 285–96. See also Loudon, *Medical Care and the General Practitioner*, pp. 208–27.

9. Records of the Plymouth Public Dispensary, Plymouth and West Devon Record Office, Annual Reports, 200/86. See also the *Journal*, 14 June 1849, p. 6; and the *Journal*, 20 September 1849, p. 6.
10. Smith, op. cit., p. 251; and Alexander, op. cit., p. 17. For greater detail see Railton, *Early Medical Services*; and M. Railton and M. Barr, *The Royal Berkshire Hospital 1839–1989* (Oxford, 1989).
11. The Army medical service is well traced in N. Cantlie, *A History of the Army Medical Department* (London, 1974). See also J. Laffin, *Surgeons in the Field* (London, 1970).
12. Nelson to Baird, 30 May 1804, quoted in C. Lloyd and J. Coulter, *Medicine and the Navy 1200–1900* (London, 1963), vol. IV, pp. 152–3.
13. The work of these pioneering physicians on behalf of seamen is well explained in C. Lloyd, *The Health of Seamen* (London, 1965); J. Laffin, *Jack Tar: The Story of the British Sailor* (London, 1969); and Laffin, *Surgeons in the Field*, pp. 99–115. See also R. E. Hughes, 'James Lind and the Cure of Scurvy: An Experimental Approach', *Medical History*, 19 (1975), pp. 342–51; I. A. Porter, 'Thomas Trotter, M.D., Naval Physician', *Medical History*, 7 (1963), pp. 155–64; and W.M. McBride, 'Normal' Medical Science and British Treatment of Sea Scurvy, 1753–75', *Journal of the History of Medicine and Allied Sciences*, 46 (1991), pp. 158–77.
14. There is a biographical sketch of Burnett by H. Rolleston, 'Sir William Burnett: The First Medical Director-General of the Royal Navy', *Journal of the Royal Naval Medical Service*, 8 (1922), pp. 1–10. The

development of the Navy's medical service is outlined in B. P. Pick, 'Medical Department of the Navy in 1838', *Journal of the Royal Naval Medical Service,* 19 (1933), pp. 241–53. Burnett's work on fever was published as *A Practical Account of the Mediterranean Fever as It Appeared in the Ships and Hospitals of His Majesty's Fleet on that Station:* 1810–13 (London, 1816).

15. Medical Officers Employed, 1 January 1849, Admiralty Records, PRO, London, ADM 105/39.
16. Smith, op. cit., p. 249. The eighteenth-century histories of Haslar and the Royal Naval Hospital are admirably chronicled in Lloyd and Coulter, *Medicine and the Navy,* vol. III, pp. 207–90. For East Stonehouse see also the outline and illustrated work by P. D. G. Pugh, 'History of the Royal Naval Hospital, Plymouth', *Journal of the Royal Naval Medical Service,* 58 (1972), pp. 78–94, 207–26; and A. Hurford, 'The Early History of Plymouth Hospital', *Journal of the Royal Naval Medical Service,* 21 (1935), pp. 40–7, 138–51, 249–52.
17. Nicolas to Burnett, 11 October 1849, ADM 97/184.
18. Expectations regarding the work of assistant-surgeons assigned to the naval hospitals were set out in Burnett to Dickson, 2 June 1846, Records of the Royal Naval Hospital, Plymouth and West Devon Record Office, Letter Book 1839–47, 1827/2.
19. Dickson and Armstrong to Burnett, 25 January 1841, Letter Book 1839–1847, 1827/2.
20. Nicolas to Baring, 24 November 1849, *Papers of Sir Francis Baring,* ING Baring, London, NP5/1/3/8.
21. Burnett to Fellowes, 5 January 1844, and Dickson to Burnett, 6 January 1844, Letter Book 1839–47, 1827/2.
22. Burnett to Fellowes, 4 January 1845, Letter Book 1839–47, 1827/2.
23. Hospital records showed that 48,452 seamen and marines were received there between 1800 and 1815, most being discharged fit for service. Cited in Hurford, op. cit., p. 42.
24. Burnett memorandum to Board of Admiralty, 31 May 1839, *Letter Books of Sir William Burnett,* ADM 105/72.
25. Minute by Burnett, 25 November 1848, on Wotton to Admiralty, 23 November 1848, ADM 97/179.
26. Rae to Baring, 19 August 1850, *Baring Papers,* NP5/1/3/9.
27. Burnett memorandum to Board of Admiralty, 9 December 1843, *Burnett Letter Books,* ADM 105/73.

4: The Advent of Cholera

1. Richardson to Burnett, 8 July 1832, ADM 97/132.
2. Logan to Burnett, 10 July 1832, ADM 97/132.
3. Parkin to Burnett, 6 July 1832, ADM 97/132.
4. Cholera in Britain in 1832 is specifically covered in Morris, *Cholera 1832*; and M. Durey, *The Return of the Plague: British Society and the Cholera 1831–2* (London, 1979). See also Poynter, *The Evolution of Medical Practice in Britain*, p. 44. Among the fullest and most informative of the tracts and pamphlets produced by medical men analysing or claiming how to bring the epidemic under control is J. Ayre, *A Report of the Method and Results of the Treatment for the Malignant Cholera* (London, 1833).
5. Property rights and legal judgments as obstacles to parliamentary legislation are discussed in G. Kearns, 'Private Property and Public Health Reform in England, 1830–1870', *Social Science and Medicine*, 26 (1988), pp. 187–99.
6. Brydone to Burnett, 8 July 1832, ADM 97/132.
7. J.A. Shepherd, *A History of the Liverpool Medical Institution* (Liverpool, 1979), p. 89.
8. A comprehensive record of the epidemic in Exeter has survived from T. Shapter, *The History of the Cholera in Exeter in 1832*, edited and with an introduction by R. Newton (London, 1971). Shapter was physician to the Exeter Dispensary. Burnett was so impressed with Shapter's study of cholera in 1832 and in 1849 that he persuaded the Board of Admiralty to buy sufficient copies to distribute to the nation's naval hospitals, marine infirmaries and dockyards. Other such accounts include J. Alderson, *A Brief Outline of the History and Progress of Cholera at Hull: With Some Remarks on the Pathology and Treatment of the Disease* (London, 1832); W. R. Clanny, *Hyperanthraxis: Or the Cholera of Sunderland* (London, 1832); R. Lorimer and J. Burton, *Observations on the History and Treatment of Cholera Asphyxia as It Has Appeared in Haddington* (Edinburgh, 1832); and J. P. Needham, *Facts and Observations Relative to the Disease Commonly Called Cholera, as It Has Recently Prevailed in the City of York* (London, 1833). See also M. C. Barnet, 'The 1832 Cholera Epidemic in York', *Medical History*, 16 (1972), pp. 27–39.
9. Ryall to Burnett, 15 September 1832, ADM 97/132 : and Gill, op. cit., p. 230.
10. Morris, *Cholera 1832*, pp. 201, 205. An indication of greater awareness

was the official investigation of London workhouses conducted in 1847 and published as *Report on the Capabilities of the Metropolitan Workhouses for the Reception and Treatment of Cholera Cases*, P.P. LI (1847–48).

11. Robinson to Austin, 7 November, 1848, MH 13/245.
12. Hobhouse to Russell, 31 August 1849, *Russell Papers*, PRO 30/22/8A.
13. Christison to Chadwick, 5 October 1848, MH 13/245.
14. Pilkington to Chadwick, 10 October 1848, MH 13/245.
15. Sutherland to General Board of Health, 24 December 1848, MH 13/245.
16. Minutes of the General Board of Health, 26 March 1849, MH 5/1.
17. Love to Fitzroy-Somerset, 5 September 1849, MH 13/249.
18. Sutherland to Chadwick, 12 October 1848, MH 13/245; likewise Alison to Chadwick, 13 March 1848, *Chadwick Papers*, 171.
19. The relative value of cholera hospitals and houses of refuge was analysed in the *Report of the General Board of Health on the Epidemic Cholera of 1848 and 1849*, P.P. XXI (1850), pp. 124–32.
20. Sheffield Union Guardians to Poor Law Board, 15 September 1849, MH 10/100.
21. Sutherland to Burton, 23 November 1849, *Burton Papers*, MS 9394.
22. Sutherland to Chadwick, 17 October 1848, MH 13/245.
23. Christison to Chadwick, 5 October 1848, MH 13/245.
24. Sutherland to Chadwick, September 1848, *Chadwick Papers*, 920.
25. Chadwick to Burton, 8 November 1850, *Burton Papers*, MS 9406.
26. The operation of the Poor Law in Scotland is discussed in A. Paterson, 'The Poor Law in Nineteenth-century Scotland', in Fraser (ed.), *The New Poor Law in the Nineteenth Century*, pp. 171–93. See also Flinn (ed.), *Report on the Sanitary Condition of the Labouring Population*, p. 72; and Englander, op. cit., pp. 47–55.
27. Sutherland to Chadwick, 15 October 1848, MH 13/245.
28. Sutherland to Chadwick, September 1848, *Chadwick Papers*, 920.
29. Bowditch to General Board of Health, 10 October 1848, MH 13/245.

5: The Local Boards of Health

1. The arrival of cholera in Plymouth was noted in the General Board of Health report on the 1848–49 cholera epidemic, P.P. XXI (1850), Appendix A, pp. 140–5.
2. The *Journal*, 14 June 1849, p. 6.

3. Cookworthy's career and family are mentioned in Gill, op. cit., p. 208; and F. A. Mayne (ed.), *British Medical Association: the Book of Plymouth* (Plymouth, 1938), p. 104. See also Jewitt, op. cit., p. 408.
4. The *Journal*, 14 June 1849, p. 4.
5. Gill, op. cit., p. 231; Jewitt, op. cit., pp. 418, 435; and M. Brayshay and V. Pointon, 'Local Politics and Public Health in Mid-Nineteenth-century Plymouth', *Medical History*, 27 (1983), p. 168.
6. Jewitt, op. cit., p. 429.
7. Odgers's report is discussed in Brayshay and Pointon, op. cit., pp. 167–9.
8. Burrows to Grey, 18 October 1848, MH 13/222.
9. Rae to Burnett, 5 July 1849, ADM 97/185.
10. The *Journal*, 19 July 1849, p. 5; and McClure to Nicolas, 27 July 1849, enclosed in Nicolas to Burnett, 27 July 1849, ADM 97/183. Further information is contained in the *Journal*, 26 July 1849, p. 5.
11. The five-fields hospital is described in the *Journal*, 9 August 1849, p. 5.
12. Milroy to Chadwick, 21 September 1853, *Chadwick Papers*, 1405.
13. McClure to Nicolas, 12 July 1849, enclosed in Admiralty to General Board of Health, 14 July 1849, MH 13/252.
14. Nicolas to Parker, 13 July 1849, enclosed in Admiralty to General Board of Health, 14 July 1849, MH 13/252.
15. A John Beer was mayor of Plymouth in 1717 and the family became an extended network of political influence. John Beer, senior, had resided in Devonport in the 1830s and been a member of the Stoke Damerel Board of Guardians. His son, John Beer, junior, a lawyer, was appointed clerk to the Devonport Improvement Commissioners in the mid-1830s, later becoming mayor of Devonport. When one of his successors died suddenly in June 1849, John Beer, junior, was again appointed mayor of Devonport until a new election could be held in November 1849. At the same time, Joseph Beer, a nephew of John Beer, senior, was secretary to the Devonport Board of Health. Joseph Beer, chemist, of Plymouth and member of the Plymouth Board of Health, Poor Law Guardian and Town Councillor, was another nephew of John Beer, senior, and either brother or cousin of John Beer, junior.
16. Nicolas to Burnett, 18 July 1849, ADM 97/182.
17. G. Milroy, *The Cholera not to be Arrested by Quarantine: A Brief Historical Sketch of the Great Epidemic of 1817, and, Its Invasions of Europe in 1831–2 and 1847 with Practical Remarks on the Treatment, Preventitive and Curative,*

of the Disease (London, 1847), with an introductory letter, Milroy to Owen, 14 December 1847. Milroy remained nominally a medical inspector for the General Board of Health until 1854, although in 1852 he was sent by the Colonial Office to investigate the 1850–51 cholera epidemic in Jamaica. His 133-page report on the island's health and sanitation was published by HMSO in 1853. In 1855 he visited the Army in the Crimea as a member of the Sanitary Commission and subsequently conducted an inspection of health in the Navy published as *The Health of the Royal Navy Considered in a Letter Addressed to the Rt. Hon. Sir John S. Pakington, Bart. M.P.* (London, 1862).

18. Milroy to Austin, 20 July 1849, MH 13/144.
19. Report of the Devonport Board of Health, 15 October 1849, Records of the Borough of Devonport, Plymouth and West Devon Record Office, Proceedings of the Council 1849–50, meeting of 9 November 1849, 1814/4.
20. Milroy to Austin, 20 July 1849, MH 13/144.
21. The *Journal*, 26 July 1849, p. 5; and the *Journal*, 9 August 1849, p. 5.
22. Nicolas to Burnett, 22 July 1849, ADM 97/183.
23. McClure to Nicolas, 24 July 1849, enclosed in Nicolas to Burnett, 25 July 1849, ADM 97/183.
24. Nicolas to Burnett, 25 July 1849, ADM 97/183.
25. Nicolas to Burnett, 27 July 1849, enclosing McClure to Nicolas, 27 July 1849, ADM 97/183.
26. The *Journal*, 2 August 1849, p. 8. Subsequent details regarding the extraordinary enquiry of 31 July 1849 are from this source.
27. Sheppard to Latimer, 31 July 1849, reproduced in the *Journal*, 2 August 1849, p. 8.
28. McClure to Nicolas, 29 July 1849, ADM 97/183.
29. Nicolas to Burnett, 29 July 1849, ADM 97/183.

6: Experiment at Noss

1. The *Journal*, 14 June 1849, p. 5.
2. The records were kept sufficiently well to have enabled an interesting piece of research on the Union's affairs to be published by R. Adair, B. Forsythe and J. Melling, 'A Danger to the Public? Disposing of Pauper Lunatics in Late-Victorian and Edwardian England: Plympton St. Mary Union and the Devon County Asylum, 1867–1914', *Medical History*, 42 (1998), pp. 1–25.

3. S. Ormerod, 'Buntingford Workhouse: The Early Years', *Hertfordshire's Past*, 28 (1990), p. 20.
4. Poor Law Board report, P.P. XXV (1849).
5. Freby and Moore to Poor Law Board, 17 July and 24 November 1849, MH 12/2467.
6. Mayne (ed.), op. cit., pp. 104–5.
7. Bowden to Nicolas, 13 June 1849, enclosed in Home Office to General Board of Health, 16 June 1849, MH 13/249.
8. Minutes of the General Board of Health, 15 June 1849, MH 5/1.
9. Yonge to Nicolas, 18 June 1849, ADM 97/182.
10. Minutes, 29 June 1849, Records of the Plympton St Mary Rural District Council, Plymouth and West Devon Record Office, Poor Law Board: Rough Minutes 1844–49, 1692/53.
11. Burnett's extensive claims were published by HMSO in a thirty–five page pamphlet, *Reports on the Solution of Chloride of Zinc: As an Agent for the Destruction of Deleterious Gases, or the Effluvia Arising from the Decomposition of Animal and Vegetable Substances; for Purifying the Wards of Hospitals or Sick Chambers; and for Preserving Anatomical Preparations* (London, 1848). He revised it for publication as a seventy-four page booklet as *Reports and Testimonials Respecting the Solution of Chloride of Zinc (Sir William Burnett's Disinfecting Fluid) as a Means of Destroying Deleterious Gases, or the Effluvia Arising from Putrid Animal and Vegetable Substance, and Preventing the Spread of Infectious Diseases; – as an Application to Ulcers with Foetid Discharges and as an Agent for Purifying Hospitals or Chambers of the Sick; and for Preserving Anatomical Preparations* (London, 1850), adding a section regarding its value in the treatment of cholera during the recent epidemic, pp. 62–74. His earlier representations to the Admiralty are contained in *Copies of Reports to the Naval Department Since last July on the Effects of Chloride of Zinc as a Disinfecting and Deodorising Agent*, P.P. LI (1847–48).
12. Burnett to Richmond, 22 January 1839, *Papers of the Duke of Richmond* (*Goodwood Papers*), West Sussex Record Office, Chichester, 1599.
13. Case to Minto, 29 April 1840, *Papers of Lord Minto*, National Library of Scotland, MS 13217 and MS 13235.
14. Milne to Burnett, 27 May 1841, *Papers of Sir Alexander Milne*, National Maritime Museum, Greenwich, MLN/166/1.
15. Burnett to Richmond, 24 December 1839, *Goodwood Papers*, 1599.
16. Burnett to Cochrane, 26 November 1847, *Papers of Sir Thomas Cochrane*, National Library of Scotland, MS 2288.

17. These experiments were recorded in P.P. LVII (1847) and LI (1847–48).
18. Auckland to Portland, 7 and 29 September 1848, *Papers of the Duke of Portland*, University Library, Nottingham, PwH 611/1–2; and PwH 616.
19. Auckland commended Portland as 'so earnest a friend to the Navy'. Auckland to Napier, 13 July 1848, *Papers of Sir Charles Napier*, British Library, London, Add. mss. 40023.
20. Portland to Baring, 19 February 1849, *Baring Papers*, NP5/1/3/8. Portland had earlier reported on initial tests in Portland to Auckland, 9 October 1848, *Portland Papers*, PwH 617.
21. G. Kearns, 'Cholera, Nuisances and Environmental Management in Islington, 1830–55', in W. F. Bynum and R. Porter (eds), *Living and Dying in London* (London, 1991), p. 106.
22. Reports in P.P. LI (1847–48).
23. Burnett to Nicolas, 5 July 1849, ADM 97/182.
24. Minutes, 6 July 1849, Plympton St Mary RDC records, Rough minutes 1844–49, 1692/53.
25. Bowden to Burnett, 12 July 1849, ADM 97/182.
26. Bowden to Nicolas, 12 July 1849, enclosed in Nicolas to Burnett, 18 July 1849, ADM 97/182.
27. Bowden to Burnett, 12 July 1849, ADM 97/182.
28. Bowden to Burnett, 14 July 1849, ADM 97/182.
29. Bowden to Nicolas, 14 July 1849, enclosed in Nicolas to Burnett, 18 July 1849, ADM 97/182.
30. Nicolas to Burnett, 19 July 1849, ADM 97/183
31. Spencer to Bowden, 22 July 1849, enclosed in Admiralty to General Board of Health, 26 July 1849, MH 13/252.
32. Bowden to Burnett, 23 July 1849, enclosed in Admiralty to General Board of Health, 26 July 1849, MH 13/252.
33. Burnett, *Reports and Testimonials Respecting the Solution of Chloride of Zinc*, pp. 64–6.

7: The Epidemic and the Royal Naval Hospital

1. Minto to Nicolas, 22 September 1838, *Minto Papers*, MS 12048G.
2. Fortescue to Minto, 23 August 1841, *Minto Papers*, MS 12057.
3. Nicolas to Aberdeen, 15 September and 15 December 1843 and 27 July 1844, *Papers of the Earl of Aberdeen*, British Library, Add. mss.

43241, 43242 and 43243 respectively. Nicolas's extensive correspondence while in the Pacific is in his Letter Book, Despatches 1842–44, N.M.M. LBK/67.

4. Memorandum by Nicolas, 16 April, 1848, ADM 97/185.
5. Memorandum by Nicolas, 27 January 1849, ADM 97/185.
6. Rae to Burnett, 5 July 1849, ADM 97/185.
7. Rae to Burnett, 20 and 26 July 1849, ADM 97/185.
8. Rae to Burnett, 23 July 1849, ADM 97/183 and 26 July 1849, ADM 97/185.
9. Rae to Burnett, 10 August 1849, ADM 97/183.
10. Director-General's List of Assistant Surgeons, 1 July 1852, ADM 105/39. Kay's death from dysentery in 1853 was a noteworthy loss to the service.
11. Millar to Burnett, 31 July 1849, ADM 97/183.
12. Nicolas to Burnett, 22 July 1849, ADM 97/183.
13. Nicolas to Burnett, 2 August 1849, ADM 97/183.
14. McClure to Burnett, 15 August 1849, enclosed in Admiralty to General Board of Health, 17 August 1849, MH 13/252.
15. Benbow to McClure, 11 August 1849, *Reports and Testimonials Respecting the Solution of Chloride of Zinc*, p. 68. Fox to McClure, 14 August 1849, is also printed here.
16. McClure to Burnett, 15 August 1849, enclosed in Admiralty to General Board of Health, 17 August 1849, MH 13/252.
17. Govett to suppliers, *Reports and Testimonials Respecting the Solution of Chloride of Zinc*, p. 70.
18. Cholera figures for the Melville hospital and the Medway towns are from Drummond to Burnett, 24 August 1849, ADM 97/183; and Stratton to Burnett, 17 September and 1 October 1849, ADM 97/184.
19. Milne to Baring, 11 and 12 September 1849, *Baring Papers*, NP5/1/3/7.
20. A contemporary account from the Haslar was published by its medical Inspector, J. Wilson, *Treatment of Cholera in the Royal Hospital, Haslar, During the Months of July and August 1849, with Remarks on the Name and Origin of the Disease* (London, 1849).
21. Rae to Burnett, 13 August 1849, ADM 97/185.

8: Litigation, the Press and the Navy

1. The *Journal*, 2 August 1849, p. 8.

2. Management Committee minutes, 7 August 1849, Records of the Plymouth Commissioners for Paving, Lighting and Watching, Plymouth and West Devon Record Office, 1609/D2.
3. The *Journal*, 9 August 1849, p. 5.
4. Gulson to Poor Law Board, 5 August 1849, MH 12/2519.
5. The *Journal*, 9 August 1849, p. 5.
6. Nicolas to Burnett, 9 August 1849, ADM 97/183.
7. Rodd to General Board of Health, 6 August 1849, reprinted in the *Journal*, 23 August 1849, p. 8.
8. The *Journal*, 9 August 1849, pp. 5, 6.
9. Proceedings in both cases were meticulously reported in the *Journal*, 16 August 1849, p. 6.
10. Nicolas to Burnett, 12 August 1849, ADM 97/183.
11. Rodd to Nicolas, 14 August 1849, ADM 174/83.
12. The *Journal*, 23 August 1849, p. 4.
13. Minute by Gulson, 19 October 1849, on Rodd to Poor Law Board, 17 October 1849, MH 12/2223.
14. Rodd to Poor Law Board, 1 January 1850, MH 12/2223.
15. Correspondence reprinted in the *Journal*, 30 August 1849, p. 4.

9: Reaching the People: Controlling the Doctors

1. The *Journal*, 23 August 1849, p. 8.
2. Grainger discussed house visiting in the General Board of Health report on the 1848–49 cholera epidemic, P.P. XXI (1850), Appendix B, pp. 145–78. Milroy was another expert who urged the benefit of early detection and treatment at home and who disparaged cholera hospitals as both expensive and detrimental to the patient. See Milroy, *The Cholera not to be Arrested by Quarantine*, p. 42.
3. Alison to Sutherland, 19 October 1848, MH 13/245; Alison to Chadwick, 13 March 1848, *Chadwick Papers*, 171.
4. Sutherland to Austin, 7 December 1848, *Chadwick Papers*, 920.
5. Sutherland's experience at Dumfries appeared in the General Board of Health report on the 1848–49 cholera epidemic, P.P. XXI (1850), Appendix A, pp. 57–70.
6. Chadwick to Ward, 24 October 1849, *Chadwick Papers*, 2055.
7. Sandon to Burnett, 11 October 1853, ADM 97/205.
8. The *Journal*, 15 November 1849, p. 7.
9. Working-class attitudes in the nineteenth century are discussed in Szreter, 'The Importance of Social Intervention', pp. 32–3; and

Morris, *Cholera 1832*, pp. 96–117. See also Smith, op. cit., p. 229; Pickstone, *Medicine and Industrial Society*, pp. 59–60; Henriques, *Before the Welfare State*, pp. 140, 148; and P. M. S. Russell, *A History of the Exeter Hospitals, 1170–1948* (Exeter, 1976), pp. 88–91.

10. Chadwick to Delane, 19 September 1849, quoted in Lewis, op. cit., p. 209.
11. Charity in nineteenth-century Britain is explored in F. K. Prochaska, *Women and Philanthropy in Nineteenth-century England* (Oxford, 1980); and M. W. Dupree, 'Family Care and Hospital Care: The 'Sick Poor' in Nineteenth-century Glasgow', *Social History of Medicine*, 6 (1993), pp. 195–211. See also Morris, *Class, Sect and Party*, pp. 161–227; and A. Summers, 'A Home from Home – Women's Philanthropic Work in the Nineteenth Century', in S. Burman (ed.), *Fit Work for Women* (New York, 1979), pp. 33–63.
12. Tenth Annual Report, 4 February 1850, 709/1.
13. Shapter, op. cit., pp. 120–9.
14. Lewis, op. cit., pp. 204–5. Similar difficulties in Liverpool are described in W. M. Frazer, *Duncan of Liverpool* (London, 1947), pp. 68–71.
15. Smith, op. cit., p. 260; and M. W. Flinn, 'Medical Services Under the New Poor Law', in Fraser (ed.), *The New Poor Law in the Nineteenth Century*, p. 56. The development of nursing in the mid-nineteenth century is more comprehensively studied in A. Summers, 'The Costs and Benefits of Caring: Nursing Charities, c.1830–c.1860', in Barry and Jones (eds), op. cit., pp. 133–48. See also S. W. F. Holloway, 'The All Saints' Sisterhood at University College Hospital, 1862–99', *Medical History*, 3 (1959), pp. 146–56.
16. Sellon's life and work at Devonport is analysed in T. J. Williams, *Priscilla Lydia Sellon: The Restorer After Three Centuries of the Religious Life in the English Church* (London, 1950). There are also references in S. Mumm, *Stolen Daughters, Virgin Mothers: Anglican Sisterhoods in Victorian Britain* (London, 1999), pp. 6–7; and M. Vicinus, *Independent Women: Work and Community for Single women 1850–1920* (London, 1985), pp. 46–89. See also C. Jones, 'Sisters of Charity and the Ailing Poor', *Social History of Medicine*, 2 (1989), pp. 339–48.
17. Various tracts attacked the Devonport Sisters, most prominently that by the Reverend James Spurrell, *Miss Sellon and the 'Sisters of Mercy': An Exposure of the Constitution, Rules, Religious Views and Practical Working of Their Society* (London, 1852); and Spurrell's *A Rejoinder to*

the Reply of the Superior of the Society of the Sisters of Mercy of Devonport and Plymouth to a Pamphlet Entitled Miss Sellon and the 'Sisters of Mercy' (London, 1852). Sellon responded with her *Reply to a Tract by the Rev. J. Spurrell Containing Certain Charges Concerning the Society of the Sisters of Mercy of Devonport and Plymouth* (London, 1852); and was supported by her father William Sellon in *Miss Sellon and the Sisters of Mercy: A Contradiction of the Alleged Acts of Cruelty Exercised by Miss Sellon and a Refutation of Certain Statements Put Forth in the Tracts of the Rev. Mr. Spurrell, Miss Campbell and Others* (London, 1852). Lydia Sellon had earlier published *A Letter Concerning the Work of the Sisters of Mercy of Devonport and Plymouth* (London, 1850). Some of this material was later collated and added to as *Letters on the Plymouth Sisters, Suggested by the Recent Pamphlets and Letters of the Rev. J. Spurrell, Miss Sellon, and the Bishop of Exeter* (London, 1852).

18. Within four years of opening in 1848 the Devonport orphanage accommodated twenty-seven girls, had room for twenty-six boys and had eight lodging houses for families. A total of 152 inhabitants lived under the rules of the foundation. It ran a girls' school with fifty pupils and an infants' school for fifty-three pupils. A further eighty-five children attended its industrial school. Additionally, its soup kitchen fed between eighty and a hundred persons daily. Details are contained in a letter from Sister Catherine to the Reverend E. Coleridge, 14 January 1852, quoted in W. M. Colles, *Sisters of Mercy, Sisters of Misery: Or Miss Sellon in the Family* (London, 1852), pp. 23–4.
19. A first-hand account of nursing in Plymouth has survived, in M. Goodman, *Experiences of an English Sister of Mercy* (London, 1862), pp. 32–54.
20. Nicolas to Burnett, 18 July 1849, ADM 97/182.
21. Chadwick to Carlisle, 5 December 1848, *Chadwick Papers*, 1055.
22. The *Journal*, 9 August 1849, p. 2.
23. The *Journal*, 20 December 1849, p. 3.
24. The *Journal*, 9 August 1849, p. 6.
25. Minutes, 17 August 1849, Plympton St Mary RDC records, Rough minutes 1844–49, 1692/53, and Smith, op. cit., p. 356.
26. The *Journal*, 23 August 1849, p. 2.
27. The *Journal*, 6 September 1849, p. 5.
28. Loudon, *Medical Care and the General Practitioner*, p. 306. For specific studies see H. Marland, 'The Medical Activities of Mid-Nineteenth-century Chemists and Druggists, with Special Reference to Wakefield

and Huddersfield', *Medical History*, 31 (1987), pp. 415–39; and J. K. Crellin, 'Pharmaceutical History and Its sources in the Wellcome Collections', *Medical History*, 11 (1967), pp. 215–27. See also S. W. F. Holloway, 'The Apothecaries' Act, 1815: A Reinterpretation', *Medical History*, 10 (1966), pp. 107–29, 221–36.

29. The *Journal*, 23 August 1849, p. 8.
30. The *Journal*, 1 November 1849, p. 2.
31. The *Journal*, 8 November 1849, p. 2.
32. Pedler to Poor Law Board, 19 May and 8 August 1849, MH 12/1367. The St Germans Union was returned as spending £7,151 on poor relief in 1848 from a total rate levy of £8,231 in the Poor Law Board report, P.P. XXV (1849).
33. The *Journal*, 6 September 1849, p. 8.
34. Minutes, 3, 10 and 17 August 1849, Plympton St Mary RDC records, Rough minutes 1844–49, 1692/53.
35. Meeting, 31 October 1849, Records of the Borough of Devonport, Watch Committee minutes 1847–54, 1814/93.

10: Conclusion

1. R. Rawlinson, *Report to the General Board of Health on a Preliminary Enquiry into the Sewerage, Drainage and Supply of Water and the Sanitary Condition of the Inhabitants of the Parliamentary Borough of Devonport in the County of Devon* (London, 1854), p. 25.
2. Minute by Gulson, 30 November 1849, on Lockyer to Poor Law Board, 27 November 1849, MH 12/2467.
3. Report of the Devonport Board of Health, 15 October 1849, 1814/4.
4. Committee of Improvement report, 11 December 1849, Records of the Plymouth Commissioners for Paving, Lighting and Watching, 1609/110.
5. Meeting, 10 July 1849, Records of the Plymouth Commissioners for Paving, Lighting and Watching, Management Committee minutes 1847–52, 1609/D2.
6. Meeting, 30 October 1849, Minutes of the Plymouth Commissioners for Paving, Lighting and Watching 1849–54, 1609/A3.
7. Report of the Devonport Board of Health, 15 October 1849, 1814/4.
8. Ibid.
9. The *Journal*, 20 September 1849, p. 5.
10. The *Journal*, 16 August 1849, p. 6.

11. Report of the Devonport Board of Health, 15 October 1849, 1814/4.
12. Rawlinson, *Report to the General Board of Health on Plymouth*, p. 73.
13. Minute by Gulson, 28 October 1850, on Mortimer to Baines, 25 October 1850, MH 12/2422.
14. Mortimer to Baines, 25 October 1850, MH 12/2422.
15. Report of the Devonport Board of Health, 15 October 1849, 1814/4.
16. The *Journal*, 22 November 1849, p. 5.
17. The *Journal*, 20 September 1849, p. 5.
18. Diary, 9 August 1853, quoted in E. Hodder, *The Life and Work of the Seventh Earl of Shaftesbury* (London, 1886), vol. II, p. 443.
19. Private correspondence enclosed in Chadwick to Russell, 29 January 1851, *Russell Papers*, PRO 30/22/9A.
20. Minutes of the General Board of Health, 17 January 1850, MH 5/2.
21. Minutes, 31 August 1849, Plympton St Mary RDC records, Rough minutes 1844–49, 1692/53.
22. Report of the Devonport Board of Health, 15 October 1849, 1814/4.
23. Mortimer to Lumley, 21 November 1850, MH 12/2422.
24. Meeting, 16 December 1851, Records of the Plymouth City Council, Plymouth and West Devon Record Office, Special Committee minutes 1851–53, 1648/X4 (199).
25. The *Journal*, 16 August 1849, p. 4.
26. Minute by Gulson, 19 October 1849, on Rodd to Poor Law Board, 17 October 1849, MH 12/2223.
27. Minutes of the General Board of Health, 16 October 1849, MH 5/2.
28. Chadwick to Carlisle, 5 October 1848, *Chadwick Papers*, 1055.
29. Chadwick to Carlisle, 10 October 1848, *Chadwick Papers*, 1055.
30. Gulson to Chadwick, 4 October 1848, *Chadwick Papers*, 907.
31. Report of the Devonport Board of Health, 15 October 1849, 1814/4.
32. Carlisle to Chadwick, 25 August 1849, *Chadwick Papers*, 1055.
33. Report of the Devonport Board of Health, 15 October 1849, 1814/4.
34. Rae to Burnett, 12 December 1849, ADM 97/185.
35. Rae to Burnett, 20 July and 23 December 1849, ADM 97/185.
36. The *Journal*, 23 August 1849, p. 2.
37. Burnett to Minto, July 1851, *Minto Papers*, MS 12068.
38. Sutherland to Burton, 27 December 1848, *Burton Papers*, MS 9393.
39. Sutherland to Burton, 23 November 1849, *Burton Papers*, MS 9394.
40. An example of this procedure is described in J. Simpson, 'A Public Health Petition: The 1848 Act and Middleton, a Township in Lancashire', *Medical History*, 5 (1961), pp. 384–91.

41. Smith, op. cit., p. 200. Brayshay and Pointon, op. cit., p. 164 and Lewis, op. cit., p. 339 give the number as 182.
42. Minutes of the General Board of Health, 21 September 1849, MH 5/2.
43. The *Journal*, 18 October 1849, p. 4.
44. Morrish to Poor Law Board, 9 March 1852, with minute by Gulson, 12 March 1852, MH 12/2422.
45. Burnard to Lumley, 23 April 1850, MH 12/2422.
46. Gulson to Baines, 8 October 1855, MH 32/29. Both new workhouses were finally opened in 1855.
47. Rawlinson, *Report to the General Board of Health on Plymouth*, p. 11. Rawlinson was also the superintending inspector who conducted the enquiry at Devonport published in 1854.
48. The story of Plymouth's adoption of the 1848 Act is well told in Brayshay and Pointon, op. cit.

Bibliography

Unpublished Material

1. *Official Papers*

(a) *In the Public Record Office, London*
ADMIRALTY RECORDS
Series:
ADM 1/
ADM 97/
ADM 105/
ADM 131/
ADM 174/
Letter Books of Sir William Burnett: ADM 105/

MINISTRY OF HEALTH RECORDS
Series:
MH 5/
MH 6/
MH 10/
MH 12/
MH 13/
MH 15/
MH 19/
MH 25/
MH 32/

(b) At the National Maritime Museum, Greenwich
Letter Book of Commodore John Toup Nicolas: LBK/67

(c) *At the Plymouth and West Devon County Record Office, Plymouth*
Records of the Plymouth City Council

Records of the Plymouth Commissioners for Paving, Lighting and Watching
Records of the Borough of Devonport
Records of the Plympton St Mary Rural District Council
Records of the South Devon and East Cornwall Hospital
Records of the Plymouth Public Dispensary
Records of the Grey School, Plymouth
Records of the Royal Naval Hospital, East Stonehouse

2. *Private Collections*

(a) *In the Public Record Office, London*
Papers of Lord John Russell

(b) *At the National Maritime Museum, Greenwich*
Papers of Admiral Sir Alexander Milne
Papers of the Earl of Minto
Papers of Sir Charles Napier
Papers of Captain Joseph Nias
Papers of Admiral Sir William Parker

(c) *In the British Library, London*
Papers of the Earl of Aberdeen
Papers of Admiral Sir Thomas Byam Martin
Papers of Sir Charles Napier

(d) *At the West Sussex Record Office, Chichester*
Papers of the Fifth Duke of Richmond (Goodwood Papers)

(e) *At ING Baring, London*
Papers of Sir Francis Baring (Northbrook Papers)

(f) *At the Berkshire Record Office, Reading*
Papers of Sir James Deans Dundas

(g) *In the University Library, Nottingham*
Papers of the Duke of Portland

(h) *At University College, London*
Papers of Sir Edwin Chadwick

(i) *In the National Library of Scotland, Edinburgh*
Papers of John Hill Burton
Papers of Admiral Sir Thomas Cochrane
Papers of George Combe
Papers of Admiral Charles Graham
Papers of Admiral Sir Alexander Milne
Papers of the Earl of Minto

(j) *At the Plymouth and West Devon County Record Office, Plymouth*
Turnbull, A., *History of the Naval Medical Service from the Earliest Dates to the Present Time* (Manuscript, 1904)

Published Material

1. *Documentary Sources*

Burnett, W., *Reports on the Solution of Chloride of Zinc: as an Agent for the Destruction of Deleterious Gases, or the Effluvia Arising from the Decomposition of Animal and Vegetable Substances; for Purifying the Wards of Hospitals or Sick Chambers; and for Preserving Anatomical Preparations* (London, 1848)

—*Reports and Testimonials Respecting the Solution of Chloride of Zinc (Sir William Burnett's Disinfecting Fluid) as a Means of Destroying Deleterious Gases, or the Effluvia Arising from Putrid Animal and Vegetable Substance, and Preventing the Spread of Infectious Diseases; – as an Application to Ulcers with Foetid Discharges and as an Agent for Purifying Hospitals or Chambers of the Sick; and for Preserving Anatomical Preparations* (London, 1850)

Chadwick, E., *Report on the Sanitary Condition of the Labouring Population of Great Britain* (1842), in D. Gladstone (ed.), *Pioneers in Social Welfare III: Edwin Chadwick: Nineteenth-century Social Reformer* (London, 1997)

Colles, W. M., *Sisters of Mercy, Sisters of Misery: Or Miss Sellon in the Family* (London, 1852)

Gladstone, D., *Pioneers in Social Welfare III: Edwin Chadwick: Nineteenth-century Social Reformer Containing Public Health, Sanitation and Its Reform Papers etc. by Edwin Chadwick* (London, 1997)

Letters on the Plymouth Sisters, Suggested by the Recent Pamphlets and Letters of the Rev. J. Spurrell, Miss Sellon and the Bishop of Exeter (London, 1852)

Lancet,

Medical Times

Navy List

Parliamentary Accounts and Papers

Plymouth and Devonport Weekly Journal

Reports by superintending inspectors to the General Board of Health: Plymouth (1853) and Devonport (1854)

Sellon, L., *A Letter Concerning the Work of the Sisters of Mercy of Devonport and Plymouth* (London, 1850)

—*Reply to a Tract by the Rev. J. Spurrell Containing Certain Charges Concerning the Society of the Sisters of Mercy of Devonport and Plymouth* (London, 1852)

Sellon, W., *Miss Sellon and the Sisters of Mercy: A Contradiction of the Alleged Acts of Cruelty Exercised by Miss Sellon and a Refutation of Certain Statements Put Forth in the Tracts of the Rev. Mr. Spurrell, Miss Campbell and Others* (London, 1852)

Spurrell, J., *Miss Sellon and the 'Sisters of Mercy': An Exposure of the Constitution, Rules, Religious Views and Practical Working of Their Society* (London, 1852)

—*A Rejoinder to the Reply of the Superior of the Society of the Sisters of Mercy of Devonport and Plymouth to a Pamphlet Entitled Miss Sellon and the 'Sisters of Mercy'* (London, 1852)

2. *Secondary Sources*

Adair, R., B. Forsythe and J. Melling, 'A Danger to the Public? Disposing of Pauper Lunatics in Late-Victorian and Edwardian England: Plympton St. Mary Union and the Devon County Asylum, 1867–1914', *Medical History*, 42 (1998), pp. 1–25

Alderson, J., *A Brief Outline of the History and Progress of Cholera at Hull: With Some Remarks on the Pathology and Treatment of the Disease* (London, 1832)

Alexander, A., *Borough Government and Politics: Reading 1835–1985* (London, 1985)

Andrews, C.T., *The First Cornish Hospital* (Penzance, 1975)

Anning, S. T., 'The Apothecaries of the General Infirmary at Leeds', *Medical History*, 5 (1961), pp. 221–38

—*The General Infirmary at Leeds: The First Hundred Years 1767–1869* (London, 1963)

—'Leeds House of Recovery', *Medical History*, 13 (1969), pp. 226–36

—'A History of Medicine in Leeds', *Proceedings of the Leeds Philosophical and Literary Society: Literary and Historical Section*, 16 (1978), pp. 203–46

Ashforth, D., 'The Urban Poor Law', in D. Fraser (ed.), *The New Poor Law in the Nineteenth Century*, pp. 128–48

—'Settlement and Removal in Urban Areas: Bradford, 1834–71', in M. E. Rose (ed.), *The Poor and the City: The English Poor Law in Its Urban Context, 1834–1914*, pp. 58–91

Ayre, J., *A Report of the Method and Results of the Treatment for the Malignant Cholera* (London, 1833)

Banks, S., 'Nineteenth-century Scandal or Twentieth-century Model? A New Look at 'Open' and 'Close' Parishes', *Economic History Review*, 41 (1988), pp. 51–73

Barber, B., 'Municipal Government in Leeds, 1835–1914', in D. Fraser (ed.), *Municipal Reform and the Industrial City*, pp. 62–110

Barnet, M. C., 'The 1832 Cholera Epidemic in York', *Medical History*, 16 (1972), pp. 27–39

Barry, J. and C. Jones (eds), *Medicine and Charity Before the Welfare State* (London, 1991)

Baugh, D. A., 'The Cost of Poor Relief in South-east England, 1790–1834', *Economic History Review*, 28 (1975), pp. 50–68

Beck, A., 'The British Medical Council and British Medical Education in the Nineteenth Century', *Bulletin of the History of Medicine*, 30 (1956), pp. 150–62

Blackden, S., 'The Board of Supervision and the Scottish Parochial Medical Service, 1845–95', *Medical History*, 30 (1986), pp. 145–72

Blaug, M., 'The Myth of the Old Poor Law and the Making of the New', *Journal of Economic History*, 23 (1963), pp. 151–84

—'The Poor Law Report Re-examined', *Journal of Economic History*, 24 (1964), pp. 229–45

Bonfield, L., R. M. Smith and K. Wrightson (eds), *The World We Have Gained: Histories of Population and Social Structure* (Oxford, 1986)

Brayshay, M. and V. Pointon, 'Local Politics and Public Health in Mid-Nineteenth-century Plymouth', *Medical History*, 27 (1983), pp. 162–78

Briggs, A., 'Cholera and Society in the Nineteenth Century', *Past and Present*, 19 (1961), pp. 76–96

Brockington, C. F., *Public Health in the Nineteenth Century* (London, 1965)

Brown, P. S., 'The Providers of Medical Treatment in Mid-Nineteenth-century Bristol', *Medical History*, 24 (1980), pp. 297–314

Burnett, W., *A Practical Account of the Mediterranean Fever as It Appeared in the Ships and Hospitals of His Majesty's Fleet on that Station 1810–1813* (London, 1816)

Bynum, W. F., *Science and the Practice of Medicine in the Nineteenth Century* (Cambridge, 1994)
Bynum, W. F. and R. Porter (eds), *Medical Fringe and Medical Orthodoxy 1750–1850* (London, 1987)
— *Living and Dying in London* (London, 1991)
Bynum, W. F., S. Lock and R. Porter (eds), *Medical Journals and Medical Knowledge* (London, 1992)
Cantlie, N., *A History of the Army Medical Department*, Vol. I (London, 1974)
Carpenter, P. B., *A History of Walsall Hospitals 1838–1998* (Walsall, 1998)
Cartwright, F., *A Social History of Medicine* (London, 1977)
Cassell, R. D., *Medical Charities, Medical Politics: The Irish Dispensary System and the Poor Law, 1836–1872* (Bury St Edmunds, 1997)
Cherry, S., 'The Hospitals and Population Growth', *Population Studies*, 34 (1980), pp. 59–75, 251–65
Chester, N., *The English Administrative System 1780–1870* (Oxford, 1981)
Clanny, W. R., *Hyperanthraxis: Or the Cholera of Sunderland* (London, 1832)
Clark, G., *A History of the Royal College of Physicians of London*, Vol. II (Oxford, 1966)
Corfield, J., 'Buntingford Workhouse: The Building of the Union Workhouse', *Hertfordshire's Past*, 28 (1990), pp. 11–19
Cowen, D., 'Liberty, Laissez-faire and Licensure in Nineteenth-century Britain', *Bulletin of the History of Medicine*, 43 (1969), pp. 30–40
Crellin, J. K., 'Pharmaceutical History and Its Sources in the Wellcome Collections', *Medical History*, 11 (1967), pp. 215–27
Crosse, V. M., *A Surgeon in the Early Nineteenth Century: The Life and Times of John Green Crosse, 1790–1850* (London, 1968)
Crowther, M. A., *The Workhouse System 1834–1929: The History of an English Social Institution* (London, 1981)
—'Paupers or Patients? Obstacles to Professionalisation in the Poor Law Medical Service before 1914', *Journal of the History of Medicine and Allied Sciences*, 39 (1984), pp. 33–54
Croxson, B., 'The Public and Private Faces of Eighteenth-century London Dispensary Charity', *Medical History*, 41 (1997) pp. 127–49
Cunningham, A. and R. French (eds), *The Medical Enlightenment of the Eighteenth Century* (Cambridge, 1990)
Cusack, M., *Five Years in a Protestant Sisterhood and Ten Years in a Catholic Convent* (London, 1869)
Daunton, M. J., *Progress and Poverty: An Economic and Social History of Britain 1700–1850* (Oxford, 1995)

—(ed.), *Charity, Self-interest and Welfare in the English Past* (London, 1996)

Digby, A., 'The Labour Market and the Continuity of Social Policy After 1834: The Case of the Eastern Counties', *Economic History Review*, 28 (1975), pp. 69–83

—'The Rural Poor Law', in D. Fraser (ed.), *The New Poor Law in the Nineteenth Century*, pp. 149–70

—*The Poor Law in Nineteenth-century England and Wales* (London, 1982)

—*Making a Medical Living: Doctors and Patients in the English Market for Medicine, 1720–1911* (Cambridge, 1994)

—*The Evolution of British General Practice 1850–1948* (Oxford, 1999)

Driver, F., *Power and Pauperism: The Workhouse System, 1834–1884* (Cambridge, 1993)

Duffy, J., 'Social Impact of Disease in the Late Nineteenth Century', in S. Jarcho (ed.), *Essays on the History of Medicine*, pp. 255–68

Dunkley, P., 'The "Hungry Forties" and the New Poor Law: A Case Study', *Historical Journal*, 17 (1974), pp. 329–46.

Dupree, M. W., 'Family Care and Hospital Care: The "Sick Poor" in Nineteenth-century Glasgow', *Social History of Medicine*, 6 (1993), pp. 195–211

Durbach, N., "They Might as Well Brand Us": Working Class Resistance to Compulsory Vaccination in Victorian England', *Social History of Medicine*, 13 (2000), pp. 45–62

Durey, M., *The Return of the Plague: British Society and the Cholera 1831–2* (London, 1979)

Edsall, N. C., 'Varieties of Radicalism: Attwood, Cobden and the Local Politics of Municipal Incorporation', *Historical Journal*, 16 (1973), pp. 93–107

Elliott, A., 'Municipal Government in Bradford in the Mid-Nineteenth Century', in D. Fraser (ed.), *Municipal Reform and the Industrial City*, pp. 112–61

Ellis, R. H. (ed.), *The Case Books of Dr. John Snow* (London, 1994)

Englander, D., *Poverty and Poor Law Reform in Britain: From Chadwick to Booth, 1984–1914* (London, 1998)

Estes, J. W., 'Naval Medicine in the Age of Sail: The Voyage of the *New York*, 1802–1803', *Bulletin of the History of Medicine*, 56 (1982), pp. 238–53

—*Naval Surgeon: Life and Death at Sea in the Age of Sail* (Canton, Massachusetts, 1998)

Evans, R. J., *Death in Hamburg: Society and Politics in the Cholera Years 1830–1910* (Oxford, 1987)

Eyler, J. M., 'William Farr on the Cholera: The Sanitarian's Disease Theory and the Statistician's Method', *Journal of the History of Medicine and Allied Sciences*, 28 (1973), pp. 79–100

—*Victorian Social Medicine: The Ideas and Methods of William Farr* (Baltimore, 1979)

Finer, S. E., *The Life and Times of Sir Edwin Chadwick* (London, 1952)

Finlayson, G., *Citizen, State and Social Welfare in Britain 1830–1990* (Oxford, 1994)

Fissell, M. E., *Patients, Power and the Poor in Eighteenth-century Bristol* (Cambridge, 1991)

Flinn, M. W., 'Medical Services Under the New Poor Law', in D. Fraser (ed.), *The New Poor Law in the Nineteenth Century*, pp. 45–66

—(ed.), *Report on the Sanitary Condition of the Labouring Population of Great Britain 1842 by Edwin Chadwick* (Edinburgh, 1965)

Forbes, T. R., 'Mortality at St. Bartholemew's Hospital, London, 1839–72', *Journal of the History of Medicine and Allied Sciences*, 38 (1983), pp. 432–49

Forsythe, B., J. Melling and R. Adair, 'The New Poor Law and the County Pauper Lunatic Asylum – the Devon Experience 1834–84', *Social History of Medicine*, 9 (1996), pp. 335–55

Fraser, D., *The Evolution of the British Welfare State: A History of Social Policy Since the Industrial Revolution* (London, 1973)

—'The Poor Law as a Political Institution', in D. Fraser, (ed.), *The New Poor Law in the Nineteenth Century*, pp. 111–27

—*Urban Politics in Victorian England: The Structures of Politics in Victorian Cities* (Leicester, 1976)

—*Power and Authority in the Victorian City* (Oxford, 1979)

—'The English Poor Law and the Origins of the British Welfare State', in W. J. Mommsen (ed.), *The Emergence of the Welfare State in Britain and Germany 1850–1950*, pp. 9–31

—(ed.), *The New Poor Law in the Nineteenth Century*, (London, 1976)

—(ed.), *Municipal Reform and the Industrial City* (Leicester, 1982)

Frazer, W. M., *Duncan of Liverpool* (London, 1947)

—*A History of English Public Health 1834–1939* (London, 1950)

French, R. and A. Wear (eds), *British Medicine in an Age of Reform* (London, 1991)

Friedenberg, Z. B., *Medicine Under Sail* (Annapolis, 2000)

Gatrell, V. A. C., 'Incorporation and the Pursuit of Liberal Hegemony in Manchester, 1790–1839', in D. Fraser (ed.), *Municipal Reform and the Industrial City*, pp. 16–60

Gill, C., *Plymouth: A New History* (London, 1993)

Gladstone, D. (ed.), *Pioneers in Social Welfare III: Edwin Chadwick: Nineteenth–century Social Reformer* (London, 1997).

Glass, D. V., *Numbering the People* (Farnborough, 1973)

Goldman, L., 'Statistics and the Science of Society in Early Victorian Britain: An Intellectual Context for the General Register Office', *Social History of Medicine*, 4 (1991), pp. 415–34

Goodman, M., *Experiences of an English Sister of Mercy* (London, 1862)

Guest-Gornall, R., 'The Warrington Dispensary Library', *Medical History*, 11 (1967), pp. 285–96

Gutchen, R., 'Local Improvements and Centralization in Nineteenth-century England', *Historical Journal*, 4 (1961), pp. 85–96

—'The Government and Misgovernment of Hitchin: The Local Board of Health 1848–1873', *Hertfordshire Past and Present*, 15 (1975/76), pp. 32–65

Hamlin, C., 'Politics and Germ Theories in Victorian Britain: The Metropolitan Water Commissions of 1867–9 and 1892–3', in R. MacLeod (ed.), *Government and Expertise: Specialists, Administrators and Professionals, 1860–1919*, pp. 110–27

—*A Science of Impurity: Water Analysis in Nineteenth-century Britain* (Bristol, 1990)

—'Pre–disposing Causes and Public Health in Early-Nineteenth-century Medical Thought', *Social History of Medicine*, 5 (1992), pp. 43–70

—*Public Health and Social Justice in the Age of Chadwick: Britain, 1800–1854* (Cambridge, 1998)

Hardy, A., 'Smallpox in London: Factors in the Decline of Disease in the Nineteenth Century', *Medical History*, 27 (1983), pp. 111–38

—'Water and the Search for Public Health in London in the Eighteenth and Nineteenth Centuries', *Medical History*, 28 (1984), pp. 250–82

—'Public Health and the Expert: The London Medical Officers of Health, 1856–1900', in R. MacLeod (ed.), *Government and Expertise: Specialists, Administrators and Professionals, 1860–1919*, pp. 128–42

—'Parish Pump to Private Pipes: London's Water Supply in the Nineteenth Century' in W. F. Bynum and R. Porter (eds), *Living and Dying in London*, pp. 76–93

—*The Epidemic Streets: Infectious Disease and the Rise of Preventive Medicine, 1856–1900* (Oxford, 1993)

—'Cholera, Quarantine and the English Preventive System, 1850–1895', *Medical History*, 37 (1993), pp. 250–69

Hennock, E. P., *Fit and Proper Persons: Ideal and Reality in Nineteenth-century Urban Government* (London, 1973)

Henriques, U., 'Bastardy and the New Poor Law', *Past and Present*, 37 (1967), pp. 103–29

—'How Cruel was the Victorian Poor Law?', *Historical Journal*, 11 (1968), pp. 365–71

—*Before the Welfare State: Social Administration in Early Industrial Britain* (London, 1979)

Higgs, E., 'Disease, Febrile Poisons, and Statistics: The Census as a Medical Survey, 1841–1911', *Social History of Medicine*, 4 (1991), pp. 465–78

Hodder, E., *The Life and Work of the Seventh Earl of Shaftesbury* (London, 1886)

Hodgkinson, R., *The Origins of the National Health Service: The Medical Services of the New Poor Law, 1834–1871* (London, 1967)

—(ed), *Public Health in the Victorian Age* (London, 1973)

Holloway, S. W. F., 'The All Saints' Sisterhood at University College Hospital, 1862–99', *Medical History*, 3 (1959), pp. 146–56

—'Medical Education in England, 1830–1858: A Sociological Analysis', *History*, 49 (1964), pp. 299–324

—'The Apothecaries' Act, 1815: A Reinterpretation', *Medical History*, 10 (1966), pp. 107–29, 221–36

Howard-Jones, N., 'Cholera Therapy in the Nineteenth Century', *Journal of the History of Medicine and Allied Sciences*, 27 (1972), pp. 373–95

Hughes, R. E., 'James Lind and the Cure of Scurvy: An Experimental Approach', *Medical History*, 19 (1975), pp. 342–51

Hurford, A., 'The Early History of Plymouth Hospital', *Journal of the Royal Naval Medical Service*, 21 (1935), pp. 40–7, 138–51, 249–52.

Jacyna, L. S. (ed.), *A Tale of Three Cities: The Correspondence of William Sharpey and Allen Thompson* (London, 1989)

Jacyna, S., '"Mr. Scott's Case": A View of London Medicine in 1825', in R. Porter (ed.), *The Popularization of Medicine 1650–1850*, pp. 252–86

Jewitt, L., *A History of Plymouth* (London, 1873)

Johnson, A. (ed.), *The Diary of Thomas Giordani Wright: Newcastle Doctor 1826–1829* (Woodbridge, Suffolk, 2001)

Jones, C., 'Sisters of Charity and the Ailing Poor', *Social History of Medicine*, 2 (1989), pp. 339–48

Kearns, G., 'Cholera and Public Health Reform in Nineteenth-century England and Wales: Interpreting the Geographical Patterns', *The Society for the Social History of Medicine*, 35 (1984), pp. 30–2

—*Urban Epidemics and Historical Geography: Cholera in London, 1848–9* (Norwich, 1985)

—*Aspects of Cholera, Society and Space in Nineteenth-century England and Wales* (University of Cambridge, PhD thesis, 1985)

—'Private Property and Public Health Reform in England, 1830–1870', *Social Science and Medicine*, 26 (1988), pp. 187–99.

—'Cholera, Nuisances and Environmental Management in Islington, 1830–55', in W. F. Bynum and R. Porter (eds), *Living and Dying in London*, pp. 94–125

Keevil, J. J., 'Leonard Gillespie, M.D., 1758–1842', *Bulletin of the History of Medicine*, 28 (1954), pp. 301–32

Keith-Lucas, *B., English Local Government in the Nineteenth and Twentieth Centuries* (London, 1977)

—*The Unreformed Local Government System* (London, 1980)

—(ed.), *The History of Local Government in England: Being a Reissue of Book I of Local Government in England by Josef Redlich and Francis W. Hirst* (London, 1970)

Kemp, P., *The British Sailor: A Social History of the Lower Deck* (London, 1970)

Kilpatrick, R., '"Living in the Light": Dispensaries, Philanthropy and Medical Reform in Late Eighteenth-century London', in A. Cunningham, and R. French, (eds), *The Medical Enlightenment of the Eighteenth Century*, pp. 254–80

Klein, R., 'Edwin Chadwick 1800–1890', in P. Barker (ed.), *Founders of the Welfare State* (London, 1984), pp. 8–16

Koven, S., 'Borderlands: Women, Voluntary Action, and Child Welfare in Britain, 1840–1914', in S. Koven and S. Michel (eds), *Mothers of a New World: Maternalist Politics and the Origins of Welfare States* (London, 1993), pp. 94–135

Laffin, J., *Jack Tar: The story of the British Sailor* (London, 1969)

—*Surgeons in the Field* (London, 1970)

Lane, J., 'Eighteenth-century Medical Practice: A Case Study of Bradford Wilmer, Surgeon of Coventry 1737–1813', *Social History of Medicine*, 3 (1990), pp. 369–86

Lawrence, S. C., 'Entrepreneurs and Private Enterprise: The Development of Medical Lecturing in London, 1775–1820', *Bulletin of the History of Medicine*, 62 (1988), pp.171–92

—'Private Enterprise and Public Interests: Medical Education and the Apothecaries' Act, 1780–1825', in R. French and A. Wear (eds), *British Medicine in an Age of Reform* (London, 1991), pp. 45–73

—*Charitable Knowledge: Hospital Pupils and Practitioners in Eighteenth-century London* (Cambridge, 1996)

Lees, L. H., 'The Survival of the Unfit: Welfare Policies and Family Maintenance in Nineteenth-century London', in P. Mandler (ed.), *The Uses of Charity: The Poor on Relief in the Nineteenth-century Metropolis*, pp. 68–91

Lewes, F., 'The G.R.O. and the Provinces in the Nineteenth Century', *Social History of Medicine*, 4 (1991), pp. 479–96

Lewis, R. A., *Edwin Chadwick and the Public Health Movement 1832–1854* (London, 1952)

Lloyd, C., *The Health of Seamen* (London, 1965)

Lloyd, C. and J. Coulter, *Medicine and the Navy 1200–1900*, Volumes III and IV (London, 1961 and 1963)

Lorimer, R. and J. Burton, *Observations on the History and Treatment of Cholera Asphyxia as It Has Appeared in Haddington* (Edinburgh, 1832)

Loudon, I. S. L., 'The Origins and Growth of the Dispensary Movement in England', *Bulletin of the History of Medicine*, 55 (1981), pp. 322–42

—'The Concept of the Family Doctor', *Bulletin of the History of Medicine*, 58 (1984), pp. 347–62

—'The Nature of Provincial Medical Practice in Eighteenth-century England', *Medical History*, 29 (1985), pp. 1–32

—*Medical Care and the General Practitioner 1750–1850* (Oxford, 1986)

Luckin, W., 'The Final Catastrophe–Cholera in London, 1866', *Medical History*, 21 (1977) pp. 32–42

McBride, W. M., '"Normal" Medical Science and British Treatment of Sea Scurvy, 1753–75', *Journal of the History of Medicine and Allied Sciences*, 46 (1991), pp. 158–77

MacDonagh, O., *Early Victorian Government 1830–1870* (London, 1977)

McDonald, J. C., 'The History of Quarantine in Britain During the Nineteenth Century', *Bulletin of the History of Medicine*, 25 (1951), pp. 22–44

McKeown, T., *The Modern Rise of Population* (London, 1976)

MacLeod, R. (ed.), *Government and Expertise: Specialists, Administrators and Professionals, 1860–1919* (Cambridge, 1988)

MacLeod, R., *Public Science and Public Policy in Victorian England* (Aldershot, 1996)

McNeil, D. R., 'Medical Care Aboard Australia-bound Convict Ships, 1786–1840', *Bulletin of the History of Medicine*, 26 (1952), pp. 117–40

Mandler, P., 'The Making of the New Poor Law *Redivivus*', *Past and Present*, 117 (1987), pp. 131–57

—(ed.), *The Uses of Charity: The Poor on Relief in the Nineteenth-century Metropolis* (Philadelphia, 1990)

Manuel, D. E., *Marshall Hall (1790–1857): Science and Medicine in Early-Victorian Society* (Atlanta, 1996)

Marland, H., *Medicine and Society in Wakefield and Huddersfield*, 1780–1870 (Cambridge, 1987)

—'The Medical Activities of Mid-Nineteenth-century Chemists and Druggists, with Special Reference to Wakefield and Huddersfield', *Medical History*, 31 (1987), pp.415–39

—'Lay and Medical Conceptions of Medical Charity During the Nineteenth century: The case of the Huddersfield General dispensary and Infirmary', in J. Barry and C. Jones (eds), *Medicine and Charity Before the Welfare State*, pp.149–71.

Marland, H. and M. Pelling (eds), *The Task of Healing: Medicine, Religion and Gender in England and the Netherlands 1450–1800* (Rotterdam, 1996)

Marshall, J. D., *The Old poor Law 1795–1834* (London, 1968)

Maurice, D., *The Marlborough Doctors* (London, 1994)

Mayne, F. A. (ed.), *The British Medical Association: The Book of Plymouth* (Plymouth, 1938)

Mazumdar, P., 'Anatomical Physiology and the Reform of Medical Education: London, 1825–1835, *Bulletin of the History of Medicine*, 57 (1983), pp. 230–46

Milroy, G., *The Cholera not to be Arrested by Quarantine: A Brief Historical Sketch of the Great Epidemic of 1817, and Its Invasions of Europe in 1831–2 and 1847 with Practical Remarks on the Treatment, Preventitive and Curative, of the Disease* (London, 1847)

—*The Health of the Royal Navy Considered in a Letter Addressed to the Rt. Hon. Sir John S. Pakington, Bart. M.P.* (London, 1862)

Mooney, G., 'Professionalization in Public Health and the Measurement of Sanitary Progress in Nineteenth-century England and Wales', *Social History of Medicine*, 10 (1997) pp. 53–78

Morris, R. J., 'Religion and Medicine: The Cholera Pamphlets of Oxford, 1832, 1849 and 1854', *Medical History*, 19 (1975), pp. 256–70

—*Cholera 1832: The Social Response to an Epidemic* (London, 1976)

—'Voluntary Societies and British Urban Elites, 1780–1850: An Analysis', *Historical Journal*, 26 (1983), pp. 95–118

—*Class, Sect and Party: The Making of the British Middle Class, Leeds 1820–1850* (Manchester, 1990)

Mumm, S., *Stolen Daughters, Virgin Mothers: Anglican Sisterhoods in Victorian Britain* (London, 1999)

—(ed.), *All Saints Sisters of the Poor: An Anglican Sisterhood in the Nineteenth Century* (Bury St. Edmunds, 2001)

Needham, J. P., *Facts and Observations Relative to the Disease Commonly Called Cholera, as It Has Recently Prevailed in the City of York* (London, 1833)

Olien, D., *Morpeth: A Victorian Public Career* (Washington, 1983)

Ormerod, S., 'Buntingford Workhouse: The Early Years', *Hertfordshire's Past,* 28 (1990), pp. 20–8

Parry, N. and J. Parry, *The Rise of the Medical Profession: A Study of Collective Social Mobilty* (London, 1976)

Paterson, A., 'The Poor Law in Nineteenth-century Scotland', in D. Fraser (ed.), *The New Poor Law in the Nineteenth Century*, pp. 171–93

Paterson, R. G., 'The Health of Towns Association in Great Britain 1844–1849', *Bulletin of the History of Medicine,* 22 (1948), pp. 373–402

Pelling, M., *Cholera, Fever and English Medicine 1825–1865* (Oxford, 1978)

Perkin, H., *The Origins of Modern English Society 1780–1880* (London, 1969)

—*The Rise of Professional Society: England Since 1880* (London, 1989)

Perry, C. B., *The Voluntary Medical Institutions of Bristol* (Bristol, 1984)

Peterson, M. J., *The Medical Profession in Mid-Victorian London* (Berkeley, 1978)

Philips, D. and R. D. Storch, *Policing Provincial England, 1829–1856: The Politics of Reform* (London, 1999)

Pick, B. P., 'Medical Department of the Navy in 1838', *Journal of the Royal Naval Medical Service,* 19 (1933), pp. 241–53

Pickstone, J. V., *Medicine and Industrial Society: A History of Hospital Development in Manchester and Its Region, 1752–1946* (Manchester, 1985)

—'Medicine in Industrial Britain: The Uses of Local Studies', *Social History of Medicine,* 2 (1989), pp. 197–203

Pickstone, J. V. and S. V. F. Butler, 'The Politics of Medicine in Manchester, 1788–1792: Hospital Reform and Public Health Services in the early Industrial City', *Medical History,* 28 (1984), pp. 227–49

Porter, I. A., 'Thomas Trotter, M.D., Naval Physician', *Medical History,* 7 (1963), pp. 155–64

Porter, R., *Doctor of Society: Thomas Beddoes and the Sick Trade in Late-Eighteenth-century England* (London, 1992)

—*Disease, Medicine and Society in England, 1550–1860* (Cambridge, 1993)

—(ed.), *Medicine in the Enlightenment* (Atlanta, 1995)

—(ed.), *Patients and Practitioners: Lay Perceptions of Medicine in Pre-industrial Society* (Cambridge, 1985)

—(ed.), *The Popularization of Medicine 1650–1850* (London, 1992)

Porter, R. and A. Wear (eds), *Problems and Methods in the History of Medicine* (London, 1987)

Poynter, F. N. L. (ed.), *The Evolution of Medical Practice in Britain* (London, 1961)

— *The Evolution of Medical Education in Britain* (London, 1966)

Prochaska, F. K., *Women and Philanthropy in Nineteenth-century England* (Oxford, 1980)

—*The Voluntary Impulse: Philanthropy in Modern Britain* (London, 1988)

Pugh, P. D. G., 'History of the Royal Naval Hospital, Plymouth', *Journal of the Royal Naval Medical Service*, 58 (1972), pp. 78–94, 207–26

Railton, M., *Early Medical Services: Berkshire and South Oxfordshire from 1740* (Chippenham, 1994)

Railton, M. and M. Barr, *The Royal Berkshire Hospital 1839–1989* (Oxford, 1989)

Risse, G. B., 'Hospital History: New Sources and Methods', in R. Porter and A. Wear (eds), *Problems and Methods in the History of Medicine*, pp. 175–203

—'Britannia Rules the Seas: The Health of Seamen, Edinburgh, 1791–1800', *Journal of the History of Medicine and Allied Sciences*, 43 (1988), pp. 426–46

Roberts, D., *Victorian Origins of the British Welfare State* (New Haven, 1960)

—'How Cruel was the Victorian Poor Law?', *Historical Journal*, 6 (1963), pp.97–107

Roberts, M. J. D., 'Head Versus Heart? Voluntary Associations and Charity Organization in England, c.1700–1850', in H. Cunningham and J. Innes (eds), *Charity, Philanthropy and Reform: From the 1690s to 1850* (London, 1998), pp.66–86

Robinson, C., *Victorian Plymouth* (Plymouth, 1991)

Rolleston, H., 'Sir William Burnett: The First Medical Director-General of the Royal Navy', *Journal of the Royal Naval Medical Service*, 8 (1922), pp.1–10

Romano, T. M., 'The Cattle Plague of 1865 and the Reception of 'The

Germ Theory' in Mid-Victorian Britain', *Journal of the History of Medicine and Allied Sciences*, 52 (1997), pp.51–80

Rose, M. E., 'The Allowance System Under the New Poor Law', *Economic History Review*, 19 (1966) pp.607–20

—*The English Poor Law 1780–1930* (Newton Abbot, 1971)

—*The Relief of Poverty, 1834–1914* (London, 1972)

—'Settlement, Removal and the New Poor Law', in D. Fraser (ed.), *The New Poor Law in the Nineteenth Century*, pp.25–44

—'The Crisis of Poor Relief in England, 1860–1890', in W. J. Mommsen, (ed.), *The Emergence of the Welfare State in Britain and Germany 1850–1950*, pp. 50–70

—(ed.), *The Poor and the City: The English Poor Law in Its Urban Context, 1834–1914* (Leicester, 1985)

Rosenberg, C. E., *The Cholera Years: The United States in 1832, 1849 and 1866* (Chicago, 1962)

—'Cholera in Nineteenth-century Europe: A Tool for Social and Economic Analysis', in C. E. Rosenberg (ed.), *Explaining Epidemics and other Studies in the History of Medicine* (Cambridge, 1992), pp. 109–21

Rosner, L., *Medical Education in the Age of Improvement: Edinburgh Students and Apprentices, 1760–1826* (Edinburgh, 1991)

Russell, P. M. G., *A History of the Exeter Hospitals, 1170–1948* (Exeter, 1976)

Shapter, T., *The History of the Cholera in Exeter in 1832*, edited and with an introduction by Robert Newton (London, 1971)

Sheard, S., 'Profit is not a Dirty Word: The Development of Public Baths and Wash-houses in Britain 1847–1915', *Social History of Medicine*, 13 (2000), pp. 63–85

Shepherd, J. A., *A History of the Liverpool Medical Institution* (Liverpool, 1979)

Simpson, J., 'A Public Health Petition: The 1848 Act and Middleton, a Township in Lancashire', *Medical History*, 5 (1961), pp. 384–91

Singer, C. and S. W. F. Holloway, 'Early Medical Education in England in Relation to the Pre-history of London University', *Medical History*, 4 (1960), pp. 1–17

Smith, F. B., *The People's Health 1830–1910* (London, 1979)

Snow, J., *On the Mode of Communication of Cholera* (London, 1849)

Stephens, L., *History of the Naval Victualling Department and Its Association with Plymouth* (Plymouth, 1996)

Summers, A., 'A Home from Home – Women's Philanthropic Work in the Nineteenth Century', in S. Burman (ed.), *Fit Work for Women* (New York, 1979), pp. 33–63

—'The Costs and Benefits of Caring: Nursing Charities, c.1830–c.1860', in J. Barry and C. Jones (eds), *Medicine and Charity Before the Welfare State*, pp. 133–48

Szreter, S., 'The Importance of Social Intervention in Britain's Mortality Decline c.1850–1914: A Re-interpretation of the Role of Public Health', *Social History of Medicine*, 1 (1988), pp. 1–37

—'Introduction: The G.R.O. and the Historians', *Social History of Medicine*, 4 (1991), pp. 401–14

—'The G.R.O. and the Public Health Movement in Britain, 1837–1914', *Social History of Medicine*, 4 (1991), pp. 435–63

Tait, W., *A History of Haslar Hospital* (Portsmouth, 1906)

Thane, P. (ed.), *The Origins of British Social Policy* (London, 1978)

Thomas, E. G., 'The Old Poor Law and Medicine', *Medical History*, 24 (1980) pp.1–19

Thompson, F. M. L., *The Rise of Respectable Society: A Social History of Victorian Britain, 1830–1900* (London, 1988)

—*The Cambridge Social History of Britain 1750–1950*, Vol. III (Cambridge, 1990)

Treble, J. H., *Urban Poverty in Britain 1830–1914* (London, 1979)

Trewin, J. C., *Portrait of Plymouth* (London, 1973)

van Zwanenberg, D., 'The Training and Careers of Those Apprenticed to Apothecaries in Suffolk 1815–1858', *Medical History*, 27 (1983), pp. 139–50

Vicinus, M., *Independent Women: Work and Community for Single Women 1850–1920* (London, 1985)

Waddington, I., *The Medical Profession in the Industrial Revolution* (Dublin, 1984)

Walvin, J., *Victorian Values* (London, 1987)

Watson, W., 'An Edinburgh Surgeon of the Crimean War – Patrick Heron Watson (1832–1907)', *Medical History*, 10 (1966) pp. 166–76

—'Thomas Robertson: Naval Surgeon, 1793–1828', *Bulletin of the History of Medicine*, 46 (1972), pp. 131–49

Wear, A. (ed.), *Medicine in Society: Historical Essays* (Cambridge, 1992)

Webb, K. A., *One of the Most Useful Charities in the City: York Dispensary 1788–1988* (York, 1988)

Webster, C. (ed.), *Biology, Medicine and Society 1840–1940* (Cambridge, 1981)

Williams, T. J., *Priscilla Lydia Sellon: The Restorer After Three Centuries of the Religious Life in the English Church* (London, 1950)

Wilson, J., *Treatment of Cholera in the Royal Hospital, Haslar, During the Months of July and August 1849, with Remarks on the Name and Origin of the Disease* (London, 1849)

Wohl, A. S., *Endangered Lives: Public Health in Victorian Britain* (London, 1983)

Wood, P., 'Finance and the Urban Poor Law: Sunderland Union, 1836–1914', in M. E. Rose (ed.), *The Poor and the City: The English Poor Law in Its Urban Context, 1834–1914* pp. 20–56.

Woods, R., 'Physician, Heal Thyself: The Health and Mortality of Victorian Doctors', *Social History of Medicine*, 9 (1996), pp. 1–30

Wrightson, K., 'The Social Order of Early Modern England: Three Approaches', in L. Bonfield, R. M. Smith and K. Wrightson (eds), *The World We Have Gained: Histories of Population and Social Structure*, pp. 177–202

Wyke, T. J., 'The Manchester and Salford Lock Hospital, 1818–1917', *Medical History*, 19 (1975), pp.73–86

Young, K. (ed.), *National Interests and Local Government* (London, 1983)

Youngson, A. J., *The Scientific Revolution in Victorian Medicine* (London, 1979)

Index

www.ingramcontent.com/pod-product-compliance
Ingram Content Group UK Ltd.
Pitfield, Milton Keynes, MK11 3LW, UK
UKHW020123290926
15471UKWH00003B/243

9 781350 17617